BACK PAIN

BACK PAIN

Diagnosis and Treatment
Using Manipulative Techniques

by

John McM. Mennell, M.D.

Special Lecturer, Department of Physical Medicine, Medical School, College of Medical Evangelists, Los Angeles, California; Physical Medicine and Rehabilitation Service, Veterans Administration Center, Los Angeles, California. Formerly Medical Director and Consultant in Physical Medicine, Woodrow Wilson Rehabilitation Center, Fishersville, Virginia, and Assistant Professor, Clinical Physical Medicine, Medical College of Virginia

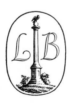

LITTLE, BROWN AND COMPANY

Boston   Toronto

To

Cecil Charles Worster-Drought, M.D.

and

Roy Michael Hoover, M.D.

with deep gratitude

Preface

The problem of the common case of backache is at least as prevalent as the problem of the common cold. But whereas the common cold if treated lasts for about a week, and if untreated lasts for about seven days, backache often undermines the economy of whole families. It is in the hope of bringing more certain alleviation to sufferers from backache that this work is being undertaken.

If some of my conclusions seem to — or do — smack of unorthodoxy, let me say only that patients in pain are little concerned with doctrinal arguments. If their pain is relieved they care little about the beliefs of him who cured them.

This work is based on my clinical experience gleaned over eighteen years of dealing with problems of the back in various countries, in many different types of patients who follow the most varied pursuits and occupations.

I have drawn freely on my previously published work on the back, and for permission to use this material I am indebted to the editors of those journals both here and abroad in which my papers have appeared. It required, however, the foresight of my friend Mr. Fred Belliveau, Manager of the Medical Book Department of Little, Brown and Company, who widely investigated the need for a more comprehensive publication, to set me the task of preparing the present volume.

Older readers will remember that I am not the first of my family to be concerned with the problems of the back. My father, the late James Beaver Mennell, M.D., of London, devoted much of his professional life and indeed many of his writings to this subject. It is difficult to follow in the footsteps of a famous father. Yet it is reassuring to conclude that most of his findings, expressed in his writings and his practice, have been tested and remain valid today. The line drawings for the section of this book which deals with the iliotibial band are taken from his book *Physical Treatment by Movement, Manipulation and Massage,* Fifth Edition, by kind permission of Mr. J. Rivers, Managing Editor, J. & A. Churchill of London, to whom I offer my thanks.

As to the neurological aspects of back pain, I make little claim to originality. Such knowledge as I have in this field I owe to my friend C. Worster-Drought, M.D., for whom and with whom I worked for eighteen months when he was senior physician at the West End Hospital for Diseases of the Nervous System in London. I cannot express my gratitude sufficiently to him.

In this country, first as Medical Director of, and then Consultant to, the Woodrow Wilson Rehabilitation Center at Fishersville, Virginia, I had the opportunity of working with patients who had supposedly reached the end of the treatment road. In suitable cases, it was found that they could still have their disabilities materially lessened, indeed sometimes removed, by the manipulative methods of treatment which are discussed in this work.

While at this center, I had the good fortune to work closely with Roy M. Hoover, M.D., of Roanoke, Virginia, who, since its inception, has been the guiding light making it the foremost rehabilitation center of its kind in the world. He has been a constant source of inspiration and encouragement to me.

To Dr. Hoover and Dr. Worster-Drought I have dedicated this work with most profound gratitude.

I wish specifically to thank for their courtesy the Editor of the *New Zealand Medical Journal* for permission to use all the illustrations and some written material from my papers, "Backache," published in Volume XLVI in 1947, and "The Intervertebral Disc and Low Backache" and "Manipulation and Treatment of Pain in the Chest," published in Volume XLVII in 1948; the Editor of the *Archives of Physical Medicine and Rehabilitation* for permission to use the illustrations of my paper "Clinical Evaluation of Low Back Pain and Its Treatment," published in February 1955; the Editor of *Clinical Orthopaedics* and the Medical Editor of J. B. Lippincott & Company for permission to use the illustrations and some of the written material from my paper "Manipulation and the Treatment of Low Back Pain," published in Volume 5 in 1955; the Managing Editor of W. B. Saunders Company for permission to use all the illustrations and some of the material prepared for the Seventh International Congress on Rheumatic Diseases as a paper, " 'Rheumatic' Symptoms Arising from the Cervical Spine and Their Treatment," abstracted in the Proceedings of the Congress in 1949; the Editor of the *Medical Annals of the District of Columbia* for permission to use the illustrations and some of the written material from my paper "Pain in Osteoarthritis — A Working Hypothesis as a Basis for Treatment," published in 1956.

Mr. A. J. C. Fisher, A.R.C.A., principal of the Elam School of Art, Auckland, New Zealand, provided all the line drawings to illustrate the examining techniques used in the cervical spine.

Many have tried to reduce these procedures to line drawings — none has succeeded so well as he.

The late L. R. Shore, M.D., made the line drawings which illustrate the examining techniques used in the thoracic spine. He was a great anatomist. I have been indebted to him ever since I became his student in medical school. These drawings were his last professional work.

Miss Audrey Tapia, secretary to F. B. Moor, M.D., Professor of Physical Medicine, College of Medical Evangelists, drew the excellent picture which is reproduced as Figure 29B.

I am especially grateful to Mr. Sal DiFede, R.P.T.A., and Mr. James Shearin, R.O.T., who modeled for many of the illustrations and who have kindly allowed us to reproduce their likenesses so frequently.

The photographic honors have to be shared by Mr. William Alwood, Mr. Charles Smith, Mr. Richard Fletcher, Mr. James Hawkins, Mr. Anthony Young, and Roger Shannon, M.D., who also provided the line drawing illustrating the effect of tendo Achillis length on posture, and to each one I wish to express my best thanks.

I wish also to express my gratitude to Mrs. Richard DeGarmo, who typed and retyped this manuscript so untiringly.

I wish also to thank those many others whose influence has matured my thoughts through the years and who, though not identified here, will understand this reference.

I wish particularly to thank my friend Robert Carney Luckey, M.D., who undertook the task of checking the professional part of this book.

For the assistance rendered by my friends, Frances Brennecke, M.D., and Thomas Wright, M.D., I am as indebted as they know.

Finally, I wish to thank C. A. H., who has spent many hours in helping to convert my original text into better English and who made me rewrite almost the whole work. But time, unfortunately, has not permitted me to incorporate in their entirety all of the many further suggestions which he has made.

J. McM. M.

Contents

BACK PAIN

1

Preamble

For many years, in a practice which has been concerned largely with patients from all walks of life who have suffered from painful joints — a majority of whom had a chief complaint of pain in the back — and who had not found relief from orthodox methods of treatment, I have used a method of evaluating and treating them which has been most satisfactory.

The method has been especially useful in relieving symptoms arising from any part of the spine which are not caused by herniated discs or other gross pathological processes. At the same time, the method of examination which I use does not fail to detect such conditions in patients, but patients with these conditions constitute a very small percentage of people who suffer from back pain. In fact, by its use, it is possible to detect and diagnose disease earlier when suitable treatment stands a better chance of being effective and will leave less permanent disability.

It is because others who have adopted these techniques have also found this to be true that I have been asked to write this presentation.

During the past fifty years there have been six major theories as to the cause of pain in the low back. Methods of treatment have been devised for each one. The sciatic nerve theory, with treatment by injection of the nerve, stretching of the nerve, and rest with analgesics and narcotics, obviously left much to be desired. The sacroiliac joint theory, with treatment by exercise, bracing, section of the iliotibial bands, forceful manipulation, and fusion of the joint, probably brought more relief to more patients, but again it obviously was not the answer to the problem. The theory that low back pain was essentially a manifestation of psychoneurosis then led the field for a short period. This was so obviously an untenable theory that it very soon fell into disrepute, though some still cling to it with blind stubbornness. Then the disc theory was suddenly accepted by the medical profession and has held its position longer than any other. The very real problem of the disc will be discussed at some length later (Chapter 11). Concurrently with this theory, the muscle spasm theory and the facet joint theory have waxed and waned, together with their varied treatments.

None of these theories ever lived up to the claims made for them by their proponents, though there was some truth to a greater or lesser degree in each of them. Even disc enucleation, which so obviously removes something, still fails far too frequently to relieve all of a patient's symptoms. It is interesting that as the fashion in diagnosis changes, the routines in treatment change very little if at all, except in the surgical approach.

Yet throughout this whole period, the pathological concept which is to be described was either known or sensed and the method of treatment has been used more or less skillfully by a few medical men and innumerable practitioners not medically qualified. The public soon came to realize that they would find greater relief more quickly and more economically from osteopathic and chiropractic treatment of their backs than they would from orthodox medical treatment. Because the original underlying pathological concepts of the osteopathic and chiropractic schools were unacceptable to orthodox medicine — and they certainly found no basis in medical pathology — the work of these groups was condemned or ignored. The diagnostic limitations of these practitioners would have been fairer grounds on which to base criticism of their methods. They, too, failed to bring lasting relief to patients more often than they should because they ignored all the structures in the back except the joints.

The changes in diagnostic fashion to which I have alluded have not been prompted by the results of any clinicopathological research. There have been no real research programs on the subject of backache. It seems that money is only available for research in the killing diseases and those crippling diseases whose disabilities are grossly obvious to the man in the street. Backache neither kills nor is painfully obvious except, perhaps, to insurance companies, whose annual payoff for claims of permanent partial back disability is probably one of their larger budgetable items.

If our nation's scientists and engineers had been as slow in their inquiries into the mysteries of outer space as our profession has been in its inquiries into the mysteries of joint spaces, our country would surely have degenerated into a second-rate power. Our profession has been rapidly losing ground to other groups who practice the healing arts in all problems concerning joint pain but particularly in the field of back pain.

This work was not supported by grants from this or that foundation. It has been made possible by the continued support of Mr. and Mrs. John Doe, who suffer unhappily from what too many professional people consider to be their psychoneuroses or compensationitis — convenient pseudodiagnoses.

Backache results in one of the greatest economic drains on

the civilized world today, not only in money but in loss of pro-
ductivity. In industry it is a major economic problem; in the
armed services it is a major personnel problem.

In 1756 that great teacher of surgery, Percivall Pott, wrote:

> I am aware that some of my readers may be inclined to charge me
> with affecting to deviate from the commonly prescribed rules; and
> to contradict opinions, which a great length of time, and a long
> succession of writers, have given sanction to.
>
> . . . *"Quae*
> *Imberbes didicere, senes*
> *perdenda fateri";*
>
> is a hard lesson sometimes to human vanity, and what requires
> some degree of candour to learn. But, on the other hand, if it
> was not now and then practiced, I know not how such an art as
> surgery (whose basis is experience) could ever be improved. . . .
> If what I have to urge is not capable of being verified and con-
> firmed by experience, it must sink to nothing; but if, upon trial, it
> shall be found by the majority (as it has been by me and some
> others) to be not only true and practicable, but highly conducive
> to the ease and benefit of the afflicted, it ought to have as much
> weight, though delivered by a living writer, as if it had proceeded
> from the remotest antiquity: its use, not its date, should give
> it value. If practitioners, since the time of Albucasis, had been
> contented with his doctrine, and never had ventured to think for
> themselves, surgery had not been what it now is, and its great
> merit would still have consisted in the multiplicity of its hot irons.

Two hundred years later all that I have to do is to change the
word "surgery" and substitute "manipulation" and these thoughts
are as true today as they were then, especially when put into
the context of caring for sufferers from back pain.

It is with a feeling of some urgency, then, that this work,
which for many will be new, is now being presented.

It is also with a sense of frustration that this work is offered,
as manipulation, whether used diagnostically or therapeutically,
is an art which is difficult to learn from the written word and

the printed illustration. It would be a pity if this presentation of the use of manipulative techniques in the diagnosis and treatment of back pain were to produce a wave of overenthusiastic clinical experimentation. The injudicious or impetuous use of manipulation can only result in failure, or even harm. Then it is only human nature to blame the procedure rather than the processor who uses it ineptly.

Further, it is putting the cart before the horse to present the subject of manipulation as used in the back without having a thorough knowledge of the subject of movement in the more easily accessible joints of the extremities. It is from study of movement in these more easily handled joints that it becomes logical to apply the same techniques to the inaccessible joints of the spine.

There is one thing in dealing with the back that makes it different from other orthopaedic problems: the cause of symptoms can rarely be attributed to a pathological condition affecting only one structure. In other systems in the body it is almost always possible to ascribe symptoms to one pathological condition. Symptoms in the back most often arise from two or more pathological conditions. The living anatomy of the back is so constructed that (1) no single segment of the vertebral column moves during normal voluntary movement without all the other segments moving; (2) the hard structures of the spine, because of the compactness of the components of the vertebral column, seldom are damaged without damage being done to the soft tissues supporting them; and (3) deviations from normal in the supports of the spine, i.e., the lower limbs, though not actually causing back symptoms may prevent their resolution until they are corrected.

The involvement of parts of the central nervous system by pathological conditions in the skeletal structures of the back may confuse the orthopaedic outlook but should be an aid in diagnosis rather than an added difficulty.

Simply, then, the back is made up of (1) bones; (2) synovial joints with their articular cartilage, synovial capsules and supporting ligaments; (3) activating and supporting muscles; (4) fascia; (5) skin and subcutaneous tissue; (6) blood vessels and nerves; (7) intervertebral discs. The back is exactly the same as any other part of the locomotor system, excepting that there are no anatomical bursae in the back, though adventitious bursae may develop.

These structures are subject to exactly the same pathological disturbances as they would be were they located in the limbs: trauma, inflammation, neoplasm, metabolic disease and congenital anomalies.

The only difficulty is that whereas in the limbs the anatomy can be handled, palpated, and specifically moved and have its individual functions tested, and the bones and joints — and, for that matter, the soft tissues — can be clearly visualized radiographically, this is not so in the back. But it is only logical to accept that structures which are identical anatomically and physiologically behave the same way and can be subject to the same kind of pathology in one site where they can be easily handled and seen as they do in another site where they cannot be easily handled and seen.

So, diagnosis of traumatic conditions and disease processes in the back may often have to be by inference, but it must always be logical. Logic in diagnosis means taking accepted pathological conditions in structures which are handled with ease in accessible parts of the body and, where similar structures are known to be in the back, postulating the same conditions there.

For instance, in considering a simple synovial joint of a limb, we all recognize that wear and tear produces changes which we call osteoarthritis. We recognize simple osteoarthritis, traumatic osteoarthritis, infective arthritis, suppurative arthritis and rheumatoid arthritis. We also commonly see traumatic synovitis and traumatic hemarthrosis. Moving from within the joint, we recognize tears and ruptures of ligaments. Next come changes in the muscles supporting and moving the joints, which include simple contusion, fibromyositis, tears and the loss of interstitial elasticity from the natural aging process or, following inflammation, scar tissue formation. I believe that these same conditions occur in the synovial joints in the back and in their supporting structures.

Muscle spasm and muscle atrophy have deliberately been omitted, as these conditions are usually secondary to primary joint dysfunction and are, therefore, effects rather than causes of pain. However, in the back, once the primary cause is eradicated, these secondary effects in themselves may become primary causes of symptoms, and so they cannot be ignored in diagnosis or treatment.

The close proximity of the spinal cord and nerve roots to structures other than the discs which may swell and produce neurological signs, i.e., the joint capsules and the ligamentum subflavum (which may hypertrophy), may be clinically confusing.

But all in all, if we remember that pathological conditions in the back produce the same symptoms and signs that the same conditions produce in the limbs, our handling of back problems will be facilitated and our conclusions more often correct.

When we recognize that there is scarcely a disease known to medicine which may not bring a patient to his doctor with a chief complaint of back pain, the importance of being able to rule out with confidence any structure in the back as being the seat of that pain becomes apparent.

Once having ruled out that the pain of which the patient complains is arising from the back itself, one can seek for a distant pathological cause which may be referring pain to the back.

As a last resort, one may consider the cause of backache to be psychosomatic. But a diagnosis of psychoneurosis should never be made in the absence of positive physical signs, among which the hippus reaction of a large pupil to light, hyperhidrosis of the palms of the hands, hyperreflexia in all four limbs with a negative Babinski sign, and diminished deep sensation in the Achilles tendons are a reliable tetrad.

Let it never be forgotten that pain which is unrelieved in spite of treatment sooner or later produces an anxiety neurosis. Such pain cannot be treated by psychological means. The psychoneurosis usually clears up spontaneously once the physical cause is removed. On the other hand it must always be remembered that neurotics may develop physical pain. Because of their pre-existing neurosis it may be much more difficult to diagnose the cause of this, but the fact that they are neurotic is no excuse not to examine them as carefully as one would anyone else.

Differential diagnosis in any field of medicine rests, in the long run, on adequate history taking, meticulous physical examination, and the ability to interpret positive physical signs elicited by clinical means. This is never more true than when dealing with problems in the back, where usual X-ray techniques show up only well-advanced pathological changes, and laboratory data show changes only when rare local diseases are present. Negative X-ray and normal laboratory findings by no means rule out local causes of back pain. Similarly, it is in back problems that skillful nursing still makes the difference between success and failure in treatment.

One must always be on the outlook for signs of systemic disease when occupied with problems of the back. The four most severe cases of back pain that I have known in practice turned out to be due to a dissecting aortic aneurysm, an epidural abscess, acute bacterial endocarditis, and lumbosacral facet joint dysfunction. In only one of these cases was there a primary orthopaedic condition underlying the symptoms. I have more than once seen patients being treated for "back strain" who have had spinal tuberculosis. I had two young patients in the Royal Air Force, one of whom was subject to proceedings for "lack of moral fiber," because his back symptoms were said to be excuses for cowardice, and the other of whom was said to be malingering with back pain; both had ankylosing spondylitis. I have been consulted over back problems whose cause has been found to be retroperitoneal sarcoma, gall bladder disease, multiple sclerosis, acute prostatitis, and gout. I have also been asked to treat people who supposedly had angina pectoris, migraine, cholecystitis, and that all-embracing diagnosis, "bursitis" of the shoulder; all of them, in fact, were having symptoms as a result of referred pain from their spinal joints.

The fascination of dealing with back problems is a never-ending source of pleasure mingled with anxiety and should be most attractive to both the undergraduate and postgraduate student. Yet in medical schools and resident training programs students look askance at anyone who is attracted by these problems and with horror when they are faced with such problems themselves. This reaction is only because they are exposed to no teaching on the subject, they are offered no method of clinical examination by which they can assess the problems, and they are not exposed to any useful method of treatment which can ever positively be said to cure these patients, except perhaps spine fusion, which they are unable to follow to its successful conclusion (fortunately, perhaps) because their curriculum passes them through orthopaedics too quickly.

No more can be said here about the more fascinating side of the differential diagnosis of backache and its wide medical interest, because this work is concerned with the diagnosis and treatment of the *simple* and *common* case of back pain. By "simple" is meant those multitudinous cases of back pain arising locally from simple trauma without gross external violence as an etiological factor, without fractures and dislocations, and not concerned with bone and joint disease, primary or secondary bone neoplasms or metabolic diseases of bone, which are relatively rare in practice.

In the following text there are three words which are frequently used, the meaning of which requires some explanation. The word *trauma* is used to signify the imparting of some abnormal force, which may be slight in its intensity, which produces some mechanical derangement in the joint or joints upon which it acts. The force is most often intrinsic and its nature is hidden from a patient's powers of external observation. It is something that the patient appreciates probably through proprioceptive sensation. The force may be extrinsic and therefore traumatic in the more accepted sense of the word. But whichever is the case, the patient's usual subjective reaction is that he has hurt his back. As "hurt" implies trauma, the word trauma is used in this very broad sense.

The word *pathology* is used in its widest sense to include the mechanical derangement or loss of function in joints affected by trauma, as well as in its more colloquial sense, referring to gross changes resulting from disease or neoplasms found in the anatomical structures which make up the back. Its use in this wider sense is acceptable if one regards as pathological anything that is not physiological.

The word *disease* is used to embrace those pathological conditions unrelated to trauma and includes the usual pyogenic, granulomatous, neoplastic and metabolic diseases which may affect the spine.

In concluding this preamble, I wish to state with emphasis that it is my experience that no man, woman, or child ever complains of back *pain* without some pathological cause or physical reason. If there is such a thing as psychoneurotic backache, the symptoms are vague and, of course, the signs which are elicited from adequate physical examination will not fit into any pattern which is normally expected when a pathological basis is present.

It is my belief that if the form of clinical examination which is advocated in this book is used, at the completion of it you can tell whether there is something wrong with the back or not, even if you do not know what is wrong. There is no shame in admitting that you do not know the cause of some disability; it is inexcusable to deny disability because you cannot recognize positive physical signs pointing to something being wrong.

Perhaps there is one thing worse than that, namely, prescribing treatment without first reaching a diagnosis compatible with the accepted tenets of anatomy and pathology.

It is because of the basic lack of teaching that the basic lack of understanding of back pain pervades our profession; and because empirical treatment is prescribed without pathological diagnosis, the public more and more take their back problems away from medical practitioners to those in other fields.

I hope that this work will help to restore patients' confidence in their medical care.

2

Movement— Dysfunction—Manipulation— Spinal Movement

Movement

All pathology in the back results in limitation of movement in that part of the spine in which it is situated. It is characteristic of pain in the back that it cannot be differentiated sufficiently by the conscious mind to determine whether it is arising from bone or joints or from the neighboring joint structures. The reflex reaction to pain in the back is splinting of the involved segment of the spine by muscle spasm.

Pain arising from any synovial joint, be it from within or from the capsule or its supporting ligaments, results in reflex muscle spasm in an attempt to prevent painful movement of the joint.

Pain arising from the intervertebral disc also evokes the reflex splinting mechanism of the supporting musculature, which interferes with, and may severely limit, interlaminar joint movement.

Pain from muscle pathology produces local muscle spasm which secondarily produces loss of movement in the joint which the muscle would normally activate.

14

Thus, for the most part, any diagnostic study of the back must depend on the physician's accurate knowledge of normal spinal movement and the astuteness of his assessment of impaired movement, especially in his determination as to whether the impairment is arising in the muscles which move the joints, in the joints in which movement takes place, or in the bones which are moved. Even then there is the large group of pathological conditions from which pain may be referred to the back. These may be suspected only if clinically there is found no local cause in the locomotor system for the impaired movement which is present.

It is characteristic that the mind cannot differentiate pain in the back from pain referred to the back from a visceral source through the visceral-somatic reflex arc. The reaction of the body remains the same, namely, splinting of the spinal segment from which the pain *apparently* is arising. A classic example of joint reaction to visceral disease is pain and impaired movement in the left shoulder, which may be the presenting symptom and sign of coronary artery disease.

In diagnosis of back conditions, it is less possible to rely on X-ray or laboratory aid than it is in other branches of medicine. I well remember two patients, one with severe pain in the low back and the other with acute pain in the thoracic spine, neither of whom showed any X-ray changes in the spine or any deviation in laboratory data, and who both died within three months of carcinomatosis, with their vertebrae riddled with metastases, the first from uterine cancer, the second from bronchogenic carcinoma. However, by adequate history taking and meticulous clinical examination these were correctly diagnosed ante mortem, though their presenting symptoms were purely orthopaedic in nature.

Conversely, another most dramatic case comes to mind of a patient who for many years had suffered from severe angina pectoris. Then, one day, an astute cardiologist satisfied both the patient and her family doctor that her heart was perfectly sound. Examination revealed gross impairment of movement in the joints of the thoracic spine between the third and sixth thoracic vertebrae. Restoration of normal movement in these joints relieved the patient's pain, which for all this time had been erroneously diagnosed as coming from within the heart instead of as referred pain in the precordial structures of the chest wall in front of the heart. The patient never complained of back pain at any time.

This example serves to remind us that pain from joint pathology may be appreciated either locally at a joint, or at any distant point or in any distant structure which shares its nerve supply with the joint. Indeed, one may postulate interference with the function of viscera as a result of referred joint pain through a somatic-visceral reflex arc. I am certain that such phenomena occur.

Though these are isolated cases, they are repeated in practice over and over again. They are chosen to emphasize that differential diagnosis in working with the back depends upon the clinical assessment of movement in the back and on the awareness of the significance of referred pain. Pain causes loss of joint movement, but loss of joint movement also causes pain.

The study of synovial joint movement has been limited for generations by the unchanging dogma of textbooks on anatomy which painstakingly describe the range of voluntary movement at each joint discussed in the text. It is very easy to accept that any gross disease process or trauma which disrupts the bony, cartilaginous, or capsular and ligamentous parts of the joint causes loss of these voluntary movements and that the joint becomes the seat of pain.

It was that great orthopaedic surgeon, Russell A. Hibbs, M.D., of New York, who propounded the somewhat trite truism that an impaired joint is a painful joint; the direct sequitur of this was the treatment of painful joints by fusion. But *restoration of normal movement* should equally relieve joint pain and in a much more desirable way. In fact this can be achieved very readily in a large majority of painful joints. The question remains, "What is normal movement?"

Any good clinician must be haunted by the fact that many patients complain of pain, for instance, in the ankle or wrist following the healing of a simple Pott's or Colles' fracture. It is a common observation that these joints are stiff and painful when the limb is taken out of plaster after the fracture is healed. The pain in the joints disappears only after the stiffness is resolved. This may occur in days or at the most two or three weeks. Yet many patients continue to suffer from pain for months and even years in spite of what is called a good return of function and in spite of the normal appearance of the joints in X-rays. In these simple fractures there is no reason to expect lasting pathology which might give rise to visible radiological changes in these joints.

These residual symptoms have then been rather thoughtlessly ascribed to mild arthritis and have been treated palliatively by salicylates and "supporting" bandages, and more recently by injection of hydrocortisone. In due course, characteristic changes of osteoarthritis appear both clinically and radiologically. Eventually the joint may be fused, with relief of pain. Yet even osteoarthritis cannot be a true diagnosis of the cause of pain. Anyone who has successfully treated pain in an osteo-arthritic joint must know that the treatment did not alter in any appreciable way the osteoarthritic changes in the joint, which to be visible radiologically must have preceded the onset of pain by months or years and will continue to be present forever.

There must be some other factor in the relationship between movement and pain. In fact, there is.

The range of voluntary movement described in anatomy texts is only part of the range of normal movement at any joint. This range of voluntary movement is entirely dependent on the integrity of a normal range of involuntary movement which I call "joint play." As in machinery, the play in all joints is well defined and without it, or with too much of it, the function of the joints becomes faulty. It must be accepted that the movements in the range of joint play individually are not under the control of the voluntary muscles, and therefore cannot be performed by deliberate muscle action. For this reason, their presence or absence can only be demonstrated by passive joint examination, and if they are absent, they can be restored only by inducing normal movement — which is manipulation. Using the voluntary muscles prevents restoration of joint play. The prescription of exercises alone can only delay this restoration when dysfunction is present.

The range of movement of joint play is most easily demonstrated both clinically and radiologically in the simplest and most easily handled joint of the body — the metacarpophalangeal joint of an index finger.

At this metacarpophalangeal joint, the range of movement described in anatomy texts is flexion, extension, abduction and adduction (which cannot be performed when the joint is flexed), and the composite movement of circumduction. Figure 1 shows the metacarpophalangeal joint at rest; Figure 2 shows the joint in flexion; and Figure 3 shows the joint in abduction. The relationship of the articular surfaces of the metacarpal bone and the phalanx should be noted and compared with the relationship of the articular surfaces of these two bones at the limits of the

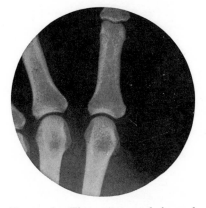

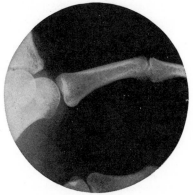

FIGURE 1. The metacarpophalangeal joint of the index finger at rest.

FIGURE 2. The metacarpophalangeal joint of the index finger in flexion.

movements of joint play which are demonstrated in Figures 4 through 7. The radial relationship of the two articulating surfaces is very constant at rest and at the limit of each voluntary movement. This relationship is very different from that which is seen at the limit of the movements of joint play.

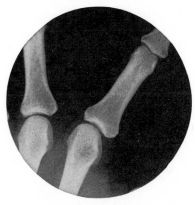

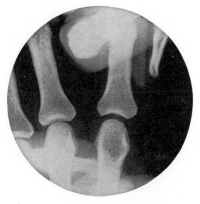

FIGURE 3. The metacarpophalangeal joint of the index finger in abduction.

FIGURE 4. The metacarpophalangeal joint of the index finger at the completion of the joint-play movement of long-axis extension.

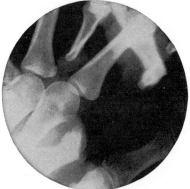

FIGURE 5A. The metacarpophalangeal joint of the index finger at the
completion of the anterior phase
of the joint-play movement of the
anteroposterior tilt.

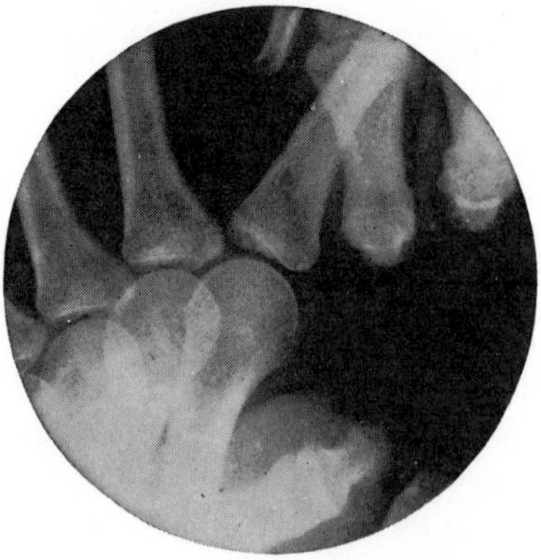

FIGURE 5B. The metacarpophalangeal joint of the index finger at the
completion of the posterior phase
of the joint-play movement of the
anteroposterior tilt.

At this metacarpophalangeal joint the movements of joint
play are:

(1) Long-axis extension. Figure 4 demonstrates the relationship of the articular surfaces of the bones, showing a wide

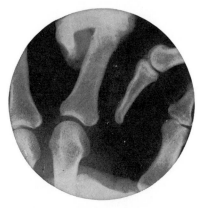

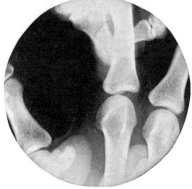

FIGURE 6. The metacarpophalangeal
joint of the index finger at the completion of the joint-play movement
of side tilt, the joint being opened on
the medial side.

FIGURE 7. The metacarpophalangeal
joint of the index finger at the
completion of the joint-play movement of rotation in the clockwise
direction.

separation of them, yet none of the soft tissue structures are stretched; only the normal slack in them is taken up. This illustration should be compared with Figure 1.

(2) Anteroposterior tilt. This is not a shearing movement but a tilting movement, opening up the joint space anteriorly and posteriorly, again without stretching any of the supporting tissues. Figure 5A shows the relationship of the articular surfaces of the bones at the limit of the anterior phase of the movement and Figure 5B shows their relationship at the limit of the posterior phase of this movement. The position of the base of the phalanx in relation to the head of the metacarpal bone should be noted in flexion (Fig. 2) and compared with their relative positions when the joint space is opened anteriorly in this movement of joint play (Fig. 5A). The performance of this joint-play movement is achieved by using the examining thumb and index finger alternately as pivot and pusher, pressing the base of the phalanx forward and backward, tilting it on the immobilized head of the metacarpal bone.

(3) Side tilt. This movement is also a dual movement in that it may be achieved both on the medial and lateral aspects of the joint. The movements are performed in the same manner as those of the anteroposterior tilt, the examining thumb and forefinger being used on each side of the base of the phalanx (instead of in front of and behind it) alternately as pivot and pusher, the base of the phalanx being mobilized on the stabilized head of the metacarpal bone. Figure 6 demonstrates the relative positions of the articular surfaces of the bones when the medial aspect of the joint space is opened up. Comparison should be made with their relative positions in abduction (Fig. 3).

(4) Rotation. In this movement the base of the phalanx is rotated on the stabilized head of the metacarpal bone both clockwise and counterclockwise with the phalanx in the rest position.

The relative position of the base of the phalanx to the head of the metacarpal bone can be appreciated when comparing rotation of joint play (Fig. 7) with the joint at rest (Fig. 1).

It will be noted that each movement of joint play is elicited by moving one articular surface on the other, which is immobilized; this is one of the cardinal rules of manipulative technique, be it a movement of clinical examination or of therapeutic implication.

It will be realized that the extent of these movements is small when compared with the extent of the voluntary movements which are dependent upon them. The fact that they are small does not mean that their importance is not great.

If you will grasp the edge of a heavy table with the hand and forearm in supination, and prepare to lift it, the upper arm is stabilized at the trunk, the elbow is flexed, the wrist is extended, the carpometacarpal joints are extended, the metacarpophalangeal joints are extended, and the interphalangeal joints are flexed. As the lifting motion starts, observe the metacarpophalangeal joint which we have been discussing. The position of the joint in its voluntary range, i.e., partial extension, is fixed, but before the table is raised at all, you can see the joint open up as the stress of the dead weight falls upon it. This movement is a mixture of the movements of joint play of long-axis traction and the anterior phase of the anteroposterior tilt, opening up the joint anteriorly. This has nothing to do with any muscle action. The muscles are occupied in stabilizing the joints for the lift. In the absence of this joint play the weight lifted would be limited by the tensile strength of the stretched joint ligaments, which certainly would rupture when lifting weight in excess of it. In fact, we can lift weights many times heavier than this because of the presence of joint play.

It is because of the movements of joint play that we rarely

suffer from fracture-dislocations around the ankle when we stub our toes or stumble, and rarely sustain fractures about the wrist when we fall on our outstretched hands, and seldom tear our ligaments when we catch onto something moving away from us. Joint play saves us a thousand times a day from bone, joint, and muscle injury; it allows the tissues around the joints to act as shock absorbers before the full brunt of the force of lifting or other force is transmitted to the ligaments and joint capsule.

Movements of joint play can be demonstrated both clinically and radiologically at every synovial joint of the extremities. If, then, other joints in the body are similar anatomically and physiologically, it is logical to assume that they also have, besides their voluntary range of movement, a range of movement of joint play. It is illogical to deny this just because these joints cannot easily be handled or conveniently visualized radiologically. In fact the synovial joints in the spine have just as specific movements of joint play as do the joints of the extremities. For normal voluntary movement they are just as dependent upon the integrity of these joint-play movements as are the extremity joints on the integrity of their movements of joint play.

Dysfunction

To clarify the difference between loss of voluntary movement, which is both subjective and objective, and the loss of movement of joint play, which is objective only, the term *dysfunction* is used to designate the loss of the involuntary movement. The loss of voluntary movement is a symptom, whereas dysfunction is a sign and when present alone is a diagnosis. It should be stressed here that dysfunction causing pain may be present without any subjective complaint of impairment of voluntary movement. The presenting symptom of dysfunction is pain either locally in a joint or at some place distant from the joint but sharing a common nerve supply.

Joint dysfunction can be caused by many conditions. Most commonly it results from trauma, disuse, postural defects, pre-existing disease, and as a result of congenital anomalies. It is also associated with bone and joint disease.

Following trauma, dysfunction is frequently associated with the hypothetical condition which we call the "joint lock." This should not be confused with the mechanical lock, or blocking of movement, which occurs in joints in which there is damage to an intra-articular fibrocartilage or meniscus as in the knee, or when there is a disc prolapse in the back. The concept of the joint lock envisages one of two things: either an unreduced sub-clinical subluxation of the joint, or a "seizing up" of its articular surfaces on one another. In the former instance, it is supposed that there is a loss of the normal anatomical relationship of the articular surfaces of the joint (probably in a torsion manner) because of the imposition of an unguarded movement upon the joint already in movement, resulting either in the synovium being pinched or a ligament being stretched abnormally. Both the synovium and the ligaments are extremely sensitive structures, having a rich nerve supply, and even minor assaults on their integrity can be very painful. The reflex reaction to capsular pain is muscle spasm. If this spasm is strong enough, the joint can be immobilized by it. Spasm initiates fatigue, which is productive of further spasm and more pain. In the latter instance, it is supposed that the articular surfaces seize up when there is simply a loss of the normal amount of lubricating synovial fluid between them following disuse. The resulting impairment of movement on attempted movement gives rise to pain which sets off the vicious circle of pain, spasm, fatigue, more spasm and more pain which results in locking of the joint.

Thus we believe the condition of the joint lock comes about. More direct unguarded force of increased severity produces dislocation. Therefore, we recognize three progressive causes of mechanical loss of function in a synovial joint resulting from trauma — (1) joint lock, (2) subluxation, and (3) total dislocation; the resulting pathological condition depends on the severity of the injury received.

Other traumatic causes which result in dysfunction are (1) immobilization of joints in plaster as part of fracture treatment, (2) immobilization of a joint as the aftertreatment of simple dislocations, and (3) the presence of intra-articular adhesions following the resolution of hemarthrosis or, if the joint has been infected, pyarthrosis.

The next four causes of dysfunction — disuse, poor posture, congenital anomalies, and pre-existing disease — should be considered together. Disuse may arise from poor exercise habits and poor posture, which may be habitual or occupational, and both may arise from the natural aging process. Pre-existing disease denotes a group of conditions which alter the architecture of the bones which form the affected joint. In the back, Scheuermann's apophysitis of adolescence, adolescent scoliosis, rickets and osteomalacia, the presence of congenital anomalies such as hemivertebrae, and even Paget's disease, senile osteoporosis, and the presence of a benign tumor in a vertebra will cause deviation of the normal anatomical relationships of the interlaminar facets to one another, producing a mechanical dysfunction even without superadded trauma. Following a crush fracture of a vertebra the architectural changes resulting alter the anatomical relationship of the interlaminar joint facets and produce dysfunction too.

Disuse, aging, and lack of exercise produce dysfunction probably by associated capsular atrophy. Ligaments, tendons, fascia,

intermuscular septa, and all interstitial connective tissue are rich
in elastic fibers in youth and health. Maintenance of elastic tissue
is dependent on activity, and once it is lost it is replaced by
fibrous tissue whose property is to contract. Fibrous tissue can
seldom be stretched without tearing and contractures remain
permanent. If a joint is not free to move, dysfunction will result.
The amount of elasticity lost in, for instance, the Achilles tendons
and iliotibial bands during a relatively short septic, toxic, or
wasting illness is remarkable. And later it will be seen how these
shortened structures affect the back and become potent causes
of back pain.

Dysfunction is, I believe, the most usual cause of pain in the
osteoarthritic joint, and for this belief there is ample clinical
support in that widely varying methods of empirical treatment
are successful in alleviating pain. For this reason, there must be
a common factor in these treatments in which lies the key to the
true nature of the cause of pain and therefore a more logical and
sure way of treatment.

The most frequent methods of treatment are (1) some sched-
ule of exercises to the muscles supporting the joint, (2) intra-
articular injection of some drug or chemical, (3) other physical
therapy which includes some form of heat, (4) some combination of the foregoing methods of treatment, (5) some recon-
structive surgery, and (6) as a last resort, joint fusion.

Each of these approaches to therapy is directed at doing something to the range of movement of the affected joint. The
prescription of exercises is the most obvious. The prescription
of fusion is equally obvious in its intent, namely, to destroy all
movement at the joint. Perhaps the most interesting treatment,
which often proves to be the most successful in relieving pain,
is that of intra-articular injection of some drug or chemical.
Lately hydrocortisone is commonly used in the United States,

but in Europe acid potassium phosphate with procaine, lactic acid with procaine, or air have been used for years. These substances have little in common with each other except the properties of either an analgesic or a cushioning effect. The large amount of injection fluid used with the lactic acid and acid potassium phosphate (hydrocortisone is used only in very small amounts), or the large volume of air which is used, certainly stretches the joint capsule as well. There is no very logical reason why any one of these substances of itself should be permanently effective. In those instances in which it is, it is probable that nature resolves some unrecognized impairment of function of the joint through an accidental unguarded movement while the joint is affected by the anesthesia or while the articular surfaces are cushioned. It is a fact that good manipulative therapy achieves relief of pain more expeditiously and with more certainty.

Impairment of joint function in osteoarthritis, therefore, merits further investigation. I feel that it is clearly the pain producer.

Impairment of joint movement in its voluntary range is, next to pain, the common presenting symptom of joint pathology and should be obvious to the examining physician. In clinical practice there can be scarcely anyone who at some time has not been confused when trying to explain the loss of voluntary movement in a joint in which no joint or muscle disorder is demonstrable by the usual clinicopathological methods. It was just because of such cases that it was first suspected that there must be more to joint movement than the mechanisms commonly described. These cases as well as cases of fracture in which there was prolonged afterpain following healing led to the search for some other cause of loss of joint function and resulted in the description of the range of movement of joint play in synovial joints.

Exactly where the pain arises is difficult to know. It probably is not in the bone, for bone pain is characteristic, being deep-seated and throbbing, and occurring especially at night, unlike the pain of joint dysfunction, which is usually sharp, occurring with movement and being relieved by rest. It cannot be in the articular cartilages of the joints because there is no nerve supply to the articular cartilage. The pain must arise in or some-where immediately around the joint capsule. The patient usually states something like "The joint feels locked." If the examining manipulative movement is tried, it will be limited and somewhat painful momentarily, and the therapeutic manipulative move-ment produces a sensation of the bones moving upon one another, and is followed by immediate freedom from symptoms. This means that there cannot be any frank intra-articular pathology such as adhesions because, in the presence of intra-articular pathology, further "trauma" inflicted on the joint, either by accident or by deliberate manipulation, always pro-duces at least a mild exacerbation of symptoms of pain and swelling.

If you lean on the dorsiflexed wrist for from 5 to 10 minutes without moving the wrist an acute pain will be produced to-gether with loss of movement in the wrist joints which lasts from minutes to hours. Voluntary movement or massage may help to speed recovery from this pain. Shaking the wrist can relieve the pain, and shaking is inexpert manipulation. However, if someone else manipulates the radio-ulna-carpal joints and the intercarpal joint, which is a composite joint, complete painless-ness is obtained immediately. The manipulation stretches each segment of the capsule of a joint to its normal limits of length and allows normal synovial fluid circulation to occur once more; the tendons, muscles, nerves, vessels, and other tissues passing over the joints are stretched too, but in no way beyond their physiological limits.

This is all that can be said about dysfunction, and it is unfortunate that its description can have no more scientific basis than that of clinical observation. Joint function cannot be studied in the cadaver because, of course, all movement is lost with death. It is possible to reproduce the voluntary range of movement in a cadaver by using considerable force, but the movements of joint play are so essentially physiological that life must be present before they can be accurately reproduced. Histopathological methods can be of no service when investigating joint function.

Manipulation

Having established an acceptable theoretical pathological entity which we call joint dysfunction, the presence of which produces the symptom of pain, the type of treatment necessary to relieve the symptom must be considered. This is manipulation.

Dysfunction, by definition, is a loss of one or more movements of an involuntary nature which occur at any synovial joint, and the performance of the voluntary movements at that joint by the action of the voluntary muscles playing upon it depends on the integrity of these involuntary movements.

Because the lost movements are primarily involuntary, they can only be restored by their being reproduced by a manipulator, who restores normal function by the use of normal movement. The normal range of movement at any joint can be described only in general terms; it can be determined only by demonstration. Thus the techniques of examination which will be described are designed to show what should be present at each normal joint. In this respect it must be remembered that every individual has his own normal range of movement, be it voluntary or in the range of joint play.

A clear distinction must always be made between examining manipulation and therapeutic manipulation. Confusion between the two is one of the reasons why manipulation has not gained the favor which it merits in medicine. I once had an intern who said: "Mennell manipulates everybody and cures nobody." In fact, during the very short time he was on my service he did not see me therapeutically manipulate anybody, but I examined everybody.

The movements of examination and therapeutic application are identical, except that in examination considerable gentleness is employed in performing each movement and each movement is stopped as soon as the patient complains of pain; in therapeutic manipulation the movement is repeated to the point of pain and then a springing thrust is added which carries the movement through the point of pain to its normal limit. Because the springing therapeutic movement is scrupulously kept within normal limits, there is usually no pain of any lasting character associated with its performance, and as a result, the joint is never traumatized further. It is not possible to perform these movements on one's own joints. The detailed techniques of manipulative movements used in examination and in therapy on the joints of the spine are, of course, described in their proper sections.

Spinal Movement

In considering movement of the synovial interlaminar and sacroiliac joints the first thing to be remembered is the type of major movement which occurs in the different areas of the spine on voluntary movement.

Normal Voluntary Movement. These voluntary movements are flexion, extension, rotation and side bending. But each part of the spine is not equally involved in all these movements by any means. However, in any voluntary movement of the spine every segment does move to a greater or lesser degree.

In flexion (forward bending or stooping) the lumbar lordosis does little more than flatten — it may achieve a mild degree of reversal; the thoracic spine flexes, markedly increasing the kyphosis; the cervical lordosis flattens and may to a small extent reverse; and at the occipito-atlantal junction a forward rocking movement occurs, this last movement being an entirely involuntary one as it cannot be specifically reproduced by voluntary muscle action.

In extension the reverse pattern occurs; there is a backward rock at the occipito-atlantal junction; the cervical spine increases its lordosis; the thoracic spine flattens; and the lumbar spine increases its lordosis.

To achieve full flexion and full extension there is a synchronous torsion through the sacroiliac joints either forward or backward. Many people still doggedly hold to the belief that there is no movement in the sacroiliac joints except in pregnant women. This belief perpetuates the greatest folly in all teaching on back problems. The falseness of it is easily demonstrated by the spreading of the posterior superior iliac spines on change of posture; this will be discussed later when considering the examination of the low back (see page 62). If further proof of the movement of the sacroiliac joints be needed, this spreading of the posterior superior iliac spines is lost when disease attacks them as in ankylosing spondylitis of adolescence (Strümpell-Marie disease) and the patient, even in the earliest stages of the disease, cannot stoop except from the hips, nor can he rotate his trunk in the sitting position without turning his whole pelvis.

In rotation, most of the movement in the back occurs in the

thoracic spine and at the occipito-atlantal and the atlanto-axial
joints, not forgetting the atlanto-odontoid joint. There is practically no rotation in the lower four or five cervical segments and
a minimal amount in the lumbar spine except at the lumbosacral junction. When the facet joints at the lumbosacral junction, instead of being vertical, are horizontal — a congenital
anomaly of the joints which I call "universal" joints — there is
an abnormal amount of rotation at this level (Fig. 8). To complete rotation there is once again a synchronous torsion movement through the sacroiliac joints, but this time there is a

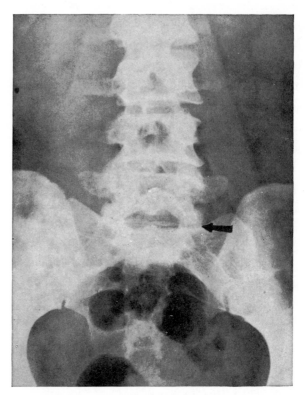

FIGURE 8.   Universal joint at the left lumbosacral junction. Normally
the joint space is vertical.

backward torsion in the joint on the side to which the rotation is made and a forward torsion on the other side, from which the rotation is made.

In side bending almost all the movement occurs in the lumbar spine and cervical spine; practically no side bending occurs in the thoracic spine.

Figure 9 (rotation) and Figure 10 (side bending) are drawn from a living subject in the sitting position. They clearly show in rotation of the trunk (Fig. 9) that the thoracic spine between A and B rotates while the lumbar spine between B and C remains

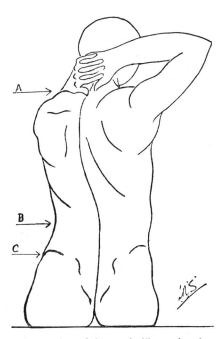

FIGURE 9.   Upright rotation of the trunk, illustrating the gross movement taking place in the three major sections of the spine. The major part of this movement takes place in the thoracic spine and at the occipital-atlas-axis joints. The synchronous forward and backward movements through the sacroiliac joints are indicated by the asymmetry of the iliac outlines. In this figure and in Figure 10, (A) indicates the level of the cervico-thoracic junction; (B) indicates the level of the thoracolumbar junction; and (C) indicates the level of the lumbosacral junction.

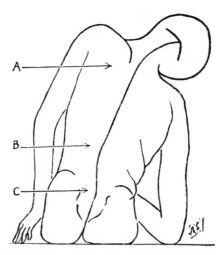

FIGURE 10.   Side bending, illustrating the gross movement taking place
in the three major sections of the spine. The major part of this movement
takes place in the cervical and lumbar spines. The line of the spinous
processes of the thoracic spine remains straight and parallel with the
middorsal line of the sacrum.

straight. The straight cervical spine is hidden by the hands. In
side bending of the trunk (Fig. 10), the lumbar and cervical
spines bend while the thoracic spine remains straight. Figures 11
and 12 show this radiographically.

Normal Joint Play. The range of movement of joint play at the
synovial joints at each intervertebral junction takes on the
characteristic of the gross voluntary movement of that part of
the spine in which the joints are situated. Whereas in any voluntary movement all the joints, including the sacroiliac joints, move,
the movements of joint play are specific at each level to each
joint on each side. It is a peculiar but interesting fact that in joint
dysfunction almost invariably a joint will be affected on only
one side of the back, and on examination, there is usually a
normal side with which to compare the abnormal side, as in
examination of the limbs.

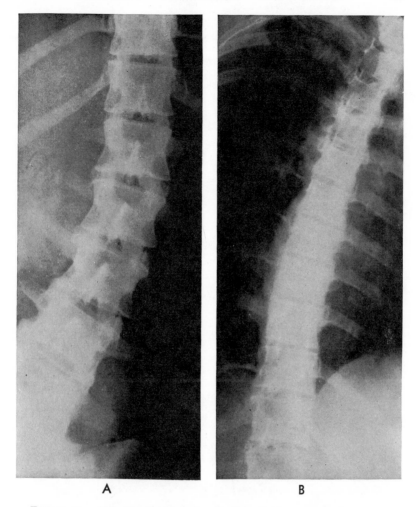

A   B

FIGURE 11. (A) The lumbar spine in the voluntary composite movement of side bending. Compare the wide range of intervertebral movement
with the lack of movement shown in Figure 12A, which was taken during
the voluntary composite movement of rotation. (B) A relative absence
of intervertebral movement in the thoracic spine during the composite
movement of side bending of the trunk is noted.

In the cervical spine, at the occipito-atlantal junction the
range of movement of joint play is long-axis extension, the
rocking movement which has been alluded to and which will be

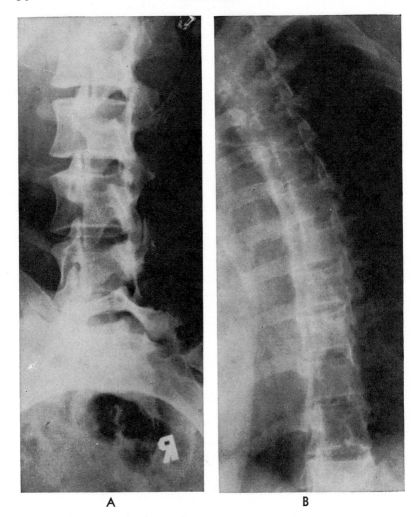

A   B

FIGURE 12. The composite movement of trunk rotation. (A) The
lumbar spine, showing the lack of movement, except at the lumbosacral
junction. (B) Illustration of the marked amount of intervertebral movement in the thoracic spine during the composite movement of trunk
rotation; this should be compared with the sparse intervertebral movement
in the thoracic spine in side bending (Fig. 11B).

discussed more fully when considering the pathology in the neck
following the so-called whiplash injury (see page 207) and

rotation. At the atlanto-axial junction there is long-axis extension and rotation. At the intervertebral levels between the axis and the seventh cervical vertebra there is long-axis extension and side bending. At the cervicothoracic junction there is long-axis extension and rotation. In addition, at each interlaminar joint in the cervical spine there is an anteroposterior glide and a side glide to the right and to the left.

In the interlaminar joints of the thoracic spine the range of movement of joint play is rotation and a backward tilting as well as a minor degree of long-axis extension. Though the costo-vertebral joints, of course, are not intervertebral, their movement of joint play has to be considered in this section. This movement is in the nature of a long-axis extension and is achieved by springing the ribs inferiorly and slightly laterally from their adjacent vertebral bodies and transverse process, thus separating the rib facets from the vertebral ones.

In the interlaminar joints of the lumbar spine the range of movement of joint play is chiefly side tilting. There is long-axis extension, a backward-tilt movement and, at the facet joints of the lumbosacral junction, a varying degree of rotation.

At the sacroiliac joints there is a forward and backward torsion which, in the range of joint play, is independent of any movement of the sacroiliac joint on the other side.

In the coccygeal joints, there is an anteroposterior tilt movement.

Finally, a special sort of movement occurs at the intervertebral body joints where there are intervertebral discs. This movement is a nonspecific universal movement in all directions, during which the nucleus pulposus is subjected to varying compression forces. The nucleus pulposus acts as a resilient shock absorber for so long as it maintains its integrity. The space-occupying property of the whole disc is the major factor in maintaining the anatomical spatial relationship between the laminar articular facets. When a disc degenerates and/or the nucleus pulposus prolapses, the laminar facet relationship may be materially altered. The resilience of the normal disc helps to maintain joint play in the interlaminar joints. When the disc degenerates and resilience is lost, joint play is lost in the interlaminar joints; then the condition of joint lock readily occurs in response to some otherwise insignificant unguarded movement. When the nucleus pulposus prolapses, it precipitates a mechanical intervertebral lock, with gross mechanical derangement in the architecture of that segment of the spine which is involved, and widespread dysfunction in the neighboring joints. The role of the intervertebral disc in back problems, the diagnosis of its prolapse and its treatment will be discussed separately (see page 177).

The clinical signs of joint dysfunction in the synovial joints of the spine are the same as those of dysfunction in the joints of the extremities, namely, impairment of movement on examination, with pain at the limit of movement. The pain is usually made worse by activity and is relieved by rest. The main difference between dysfunction in any joint of the spine and dysfunction in a joint of an extremity is that in the spine there is such an intimacy in the interaction of each spinal segment that the neighboring joints to that in which there is primary dysfunction show a degree of dysfunction also.

The examining techniques to be described illustrate the extent of movement which should be present in a normal subject. The range of movement in the joints on each side of the spine should be the same.

When examining a patient to elicit signs of dysfunction, it is the limitation of movement in any of these joints which has to be detected and assessed.

3

History Taking

In this work we are not primarily concerned with the patient who has sustained severe injury from external trauma from an accident. These patients are usually well taken care of initially and their treatment will not be commented upon here.

This work is concerned with those patients who complain of residual pain from such accidental external violence, and particularly with those who suffer from acute back pain following some stupidly trivial episode or even from no apparent cause.

There are few conditions which make a patient seek medical aid in which the history plays a more important role in diagnosis than back pain.

Past History

As in all history taking, it is important to ascertain the patient's age, occupation, marital status, and if a woman, whether she has had children and whether she has had any miscarriages or stillbirths. The age is of importance because certain specific back problems occur in certain age groups. An obvious example of this is that osteoporosis senilis does not usually occur before the fifth decade of life. The occupation is important because certain things happen to people who do heavy manual work that do not happen to people whose occupations are sedentary. Also

39

the questions of whether the patient works in a draft or in an air-conditioned office and whether he has to drive far to work or stand in bumpy public buses may give important information. When inquiring about a patient's occupation it is well to remember to ask about his spare-time occupations as well.

Inquiry as to the marital status may pave the way to later information. For instance, a patient may persist in denying any knowledge of how a pain started rather than admit that its onset was during sexual intercourse. Such inquiry may also conveniently lead the way to questions regarding venereal disease. Both syphilis and gonorrhea may produce violent back pain: the former as part of a tabetic crisis; the latter as the result of acute prostatitis or salpingitis, producing infective spondylitis. The history of stillbirths may suggest venereal disease, and miscarriages may suggest some pelvic pathology producing referred back symptoms or hormonal imbalance that might be giving rise to osteoporosis.

The family history may suggest congenital anomalies which may be passed down through the generations. The familial environment may be contributory. Some of the rarer congenital and familial musculoskeletal diseases may be unmasked by the family history. A family history of tuberculosis may be important.

The past history of the patient is of considerable importance. The history of any accidents should be noted; also any previous attacks of back pain should be studied at length. A previous history of back pain in adolescence means something very different from a previous history of back pain as an adult. If the back pain dates back to an obstetrical delivery, it is important to know whether the onset was during labor or in the postpartum period, i.e., during the stress of activity or during the involution of the pelvic joints. A past history of venereal disease, as already mentioned, must be inquired for. The nature of past illnesses must be determined and the nature and duration of any operative procedures should be noted. A past history of heart trouble in childhood, chorea or St. Vitus dance, a history of allergies, asthma, migraine and hay fever may all have a bearing on present back pain. An inquiry should be made as to whether the patient ever drank raw milk or ate uncooked meat or whether he has ever suffered from pyrexia of unknown origin. Travel abroad should be noted. I always ask whether the patient has previously consulted an osteopath or chiropractor and whether he was helped by the manipulative treatment, and how long any relief lasted.

Present Complaint

In considering the history of the present complaint a general system review must always be undertaken. I always run through the following routine, asking (1) whether the patient has headaches, sore throats, any bad teeth, or cough; (2) whether he complains of any indigestion, nausea or vomiting or bowel trouble; what his weight is, and whether he is gaining or losing; (3) whether there is any unusual amount of perspiration and if so, does it occur at any particular time; and (4) does he have any trouble urinating. Then I ask (5) about his smoking and drinking habits and what his daily fluid intake is. Finally I ask (6) whether he has any other aches or pain in any other joints or other parts of his body, whether he has noticed any temperature changes in his extremities or noted any change in his sex urges. If the patient is a woman, she is asked whether her periods are normal, and if the periods have ceased, whether she has had any loss or discharge from the vagina since.

The history of the present back pain is then taken. The first questions concern the duration of symptoms and the general locale of the pain; whether it is central or one-sided; whether it is acute or chronic, intermittent or constant.

Onset of Pain. The next question concerns the mode of onset. A description of its precise location and its exact time and mode of onset is often the most enlightening part of the history and may clearly point the way to a diagnosis. But however suggestive a history may be, no short cuts in the complete clinical examination are permissible, as the history of onset may be the most misleading part of the whole examination of the patient. An example involving a man who was a personal acquaintance, but not one of my patients, will underscore this warning. He bent down to put the family cat out before going to bed. On straightening up he stated that something seemed to catch in his back, producing acute pain, and he was unable to stand up straight. Up to this moment he was perfectly well; he had no previous back pain and his system review was negative. His X-ray findings were also negative. This history of onset is perfect for joint dysfunction at the lumbosacral junction or in one of the sacroiliac joints. Routine orthodox treatment for "back strain" by bed rest and Buck's traction did not bring him expected relief. After 10 days he was subjected to an exploratory laminectomy. No disc prolapse was found. He had a rapid downhill course and was dead in 2 months with carcinomatosis from a primary bronchogenic tumor.

There are two usual modes of onset, one sudden, the other insidious. "Insidious" is used to denote the onset of pain without any recognized precipitating movement or other traumatic factor. "Sudden" is used to denote the onset of pain during movement.

The sudden onset of pain may be during the performance of some trivial action, such as doing up a shoe lace, picking a book up off the floor, missing a golf shot, or fooling around when swimming. In the neck it may occur suddenly while brushing the teeth, putting on a shirt or combing the hair. In the thoracic spine it may occur when coughing or sneezing. The onset of pain is often associated with an immediate inability to move the affected part of the back. Frequently the patient explains that he was doing one of these simple things and that something distracted him, causing him to start to do something else, such as twist around to look behind him. Thus he subjects his joints to an unguarded movement during the performance of an otherwise normal voluntary movement. This is the type of history commonly associated with an interlaminar joint lock or sacroiliac joint subluxation.

More obviously the patient may give a history of a "whip-lash" type of injury or a mild fall, or an awkward landing after a small jump.

The sudden onset of pain while lifting a heavy object may result in what the patient describes as something catching or locking in the back, which again suggests a synovial joint injury due to unskilled lifting. The patient may, however, say that something seemed to tear in his back; then a muscle injury may be suspected.

A sneeze when a patient is in an unstable position, such as stooping to pick up a present from underneath a Christmas tree, may be sufficient to prolapse a nucleus pulposus through an already weakened annulus fibrosus. Lifting a heavy object under cramped conditions may do the same thing.

One has to try to visualize what is likely to happen within the back as a result of the strain imposed upon it which pre-cipitates the pain. This, after all, is what one does when assessing an injury to an extremity, but somehow it is easier to visualize this when it happens to something that can be seen and handled

than when it occurs in that dark mysterious unexplored area —
the back.

Pain of insidious onset may be acute or chronic in nature.
The insidious onset of chronic back pain should direct one's
thoughts toward bone or joint disease, or neoplasms in the
spine, or to distant pathology from which pain is referred to
the back.

The insidious onset of acute pain may indicate the onset of
systemic disease such as influenza. It may herald an epidural
abscess. It may be the presenting symptom of visceral disease,
such as cholecystitis, appendicitis, coronary artery occlusion or
a tabetic crisis.

Osteomyelitis may have an acute insidious onset if the cause
is a pyogenic organism, or a chronic insidious onset if the in-
fecting organism is one of the *Salmonella* group.

Nature of Pain. After determining the mode of onset of the
pain, attention is directed toward the nature of the pain and
what, if anything, may make it better or worse.

The question which gives rise to one of the most revealing
answers is, what effect does rest have on the pain? The question
is best couched in the words: "What is the pain like when you
wake in the morning?" thus avoiding a direct leading question.
The pain of bone and joint disease and muscle injury is not much
improved by rest and the back stiffens with rest in these conditions. The patient usually says that after being up and about for
an hour or so he feels much better. At the end of the day there
is a worsening of symptoms.

Pain from joint dysfunction improves with, and may be relieved by, rest, but after the patient has been up and about for
twenty minutes or so the pain returns and worsens toward the
end of the day.

Night pain in the back is characteristic of bone neoplasms, as it is elsewhere in the skeleton.

Various activities, or the assumption of certain postures, may either improve or worsen the patient's pain. It is surprising how constant are the tricks which patients discover to ease the pain from various common causes. For instance, wearing a tight belt around the pelvis or wearing a tight girdle eases the pain of sacroiliac joint dysfunction. The semistooped position adopted when ironing or washing dishes aggravates lumbosacral joint dysfunction, and relief can be obtained by sitting on a high stool to do these things. It is not especially what aggravates the pain that matters in the history, but rather the interpretation of what is happening during the activities which worsen the pain that is of significance. The information gained from the history does not result so much from conscious thought process as from unconscious association nudging a memory process built up from experience.

Location of Pain. Finally, questions regarding the location of the seat of the pain and its radiation, if any, remain to be asked. Again, the examiner must not be misled by the presence of radiating pain. It by no means specifically indicates the presence of radiculitis. More commonly it indicates pain referred along the course of the nerve which supplies the joint in which the underlying pathology will be found. A history of pain starting in the low back and radiating all the way up the back into the head, which at face value sounds bizarre and unlikely, should not give rise to too much doubtful speculation when it is remembered that the muscular support of the back relays from occiput to sacrum. Muscle spasm and fatigue may thus be relayed the length of the spine, producing secondary joint dysfunction at any level, and therefore widely distributed symptoms.

Pain on one side of the back is likely to indicate simple traumatic joint pathology, such as joint dysfunction, whereas pain on both sides of the back is likely to signify bone or joint disease. Disc pathology may give rise to unilateral or bilateral symptoms.

4

Examination— General Considerations

The examination of each part of the spine involves the use of certain basic principles common to all three areas, besides the specific techniques used in each separate area. It is convenient to consider those parts of technique which are common to the back as a whole before discussing detailed local techniques. The reader is asked to remember these general considerations as he reads each topographical chapter.

The examination of the back is not confined to the bones and joints; neither are the local causes of pain confined to them. The more common conditions which may coexist with and complicate the mechanical problems of the back — or which, by themselves, may be the cause of pain in the back — are discussed in Chapters 10 through 12. In all back problems, the patient's temperature should be taken.

It should be unnecessary to remind the reader that a patient should be adequately disrobed for any examination. This means that for back examination the patient should be stripped of all clothing and draped in an examining gown which is open at the back. The patient must always be examined in a good light which does not throw shadows on the back.

Any part of the back must be examined first at rest, then in voluntary movement, and lastly by passive movement. General deviations from the normal curves, i.e., cervical lordosis, thoracic kyphosis and lumbar lordosis, should be noted. It should be remembered that nobody can alter the contour of these curves either generally or segmentally (that is, locally, involving three or four vertebrae) without changing his stance, unless there is pre-existing neuromuscular disease or congenital anomaly.

If local segmental flattening or scoliosis is noted, the causative pathology should probably be sought for in those areas.

The iliac crests are normally level. Nobody can alter the level of the iliac crests voluntarily without changing his stance. So, if one iliac crest is higher than the other, this should direct attention to the low back as the probable site of pathology.

Every spinal segment should move smoothly and synchronously. If there appears to be more or less movement at one junction than at any of the others, it is in this area that pathology should be suspected.

The voluntary movements of side bending and backward bending in the standing position are not used in the method of examination to be described. They produce pain to a greater or lesser degree in a normal back and they are scarcely normal movements: at least they are not commonly used in everyday living. No abnormal movement should ever be used in any part of a clinical examination.

In a back in which there is dysfunction, the voluntary range of movement is limited, though this limitation is both less and more localized on passive examination. When the examination for joint play is made, the loss of movement may be found to involve only one joint and will be characterized by pain which occurs at the moment an attempt is made to perform the joint-play movement.

Neurological Examination

In looking for any neurological complication of back pain, the reflexes, motor power, and sensation in the area being examined must be checked. Though too much reliance cannot be placed on neurological signs in the determination of the level of pathology in the spine, the presence of positive signs must never be overlooked. The reactions of the pupils to light and accommodation should be noted, and the plantar reflexes should be examined.

Then too, any area which derives its nerve supply from that part of the spine which is under consideration must be examined. For instance, an examination of the lumbar spine is incomplete unless the abdomen and legs are examined. An examination of the thoracic spine is incomplete unless the arms, chest wall, and abdomen are examined. An examination of the cervical spine is incomplete unless the cranial nerves, arms and upper thorax are examined.

General Examination

The usual clinical examination of the viscera which might be involved, by way of the relative visceral-somatic reflex arcs in the area of the back being examined, must be undertaken to ascertain whether the pain in the back might be referred from these sources. So, an examination of a patient with low back pain is incomplete unless a rectal examination, and if necessary, a pelvic examination, as well as the general abdominal examination are carried out. An examination of the lungs and heart must be undertaken together with an examination of the viscera of the abdomen in patients with thoracic spine pain. An examination of the lungs and upper mediastinum and of the eyes, ears, nose and throat should accompany an examination of patients with cervical spine pain.

Circulation. The state of the circulation of the extremities must be noted when examination of the limbs is appropriate to the area of the spine under review.

Focus of Infection. When a focus of infection is being sought, every system of the body must be reviewed by examination, regardless of what part of the spine is involved symptomatically.

Stooping. There are two useful clinical generalizations which are often helpful. First, when a patient bends forward, even though the movement may be very restricted, the manner in which he recovers the upright position is very revealing. If he straightens up smoothly, a traumatic condition should be suspected. If, on the other hand, he straightens up in a tortuous manner or with assistance, by climbing up his legs with his hands, bone or joint disease should be strongly suspected in the absence of some pathological condition in the muscles.

Abdominal and Back Pain. Second, when a patient complains of both back pain and abdominal pain, the pathology will probably be found in the abdomen if the level of both pains is the same; whereas, if the level of the abdominal pain is lower than the level of the back pain, the pathology will probably be in the back. This, of course, is because the segmental nerve distribution in the lower half of the body courses caudally from its spinal cord segment.

Percussion. Percussion over a vertebra provides useful clinical information, but only the vertebrae of the thoracic and lumbar spines can conveniently be percussed in examination. Each vertebra can be more accurately hit if percussion is done when the patient is bent forward. Acute pain on percussion, which immediately disappears, suggests the presence of traumatic joint pathology, because the percussive force jars the joints. A dull pain of a throbbing nature, which slowly disappears, suggests a fracture or bone disease or neoplasm, as it does in any other part of the skeleton.

Localization. One of the most important parts of examination of any part of the back is the localization by the patient, using one finger, of the place which he feels is the seat of his pain. If he points to an area beneath which, anatomically, there is only muscle, then muscle pathology must be suspected. If he points to a spot over an intervertebral junction, then the joints or a disc may be suspect. If he points over a vertebral body, bone disease may be suspected. If he points over one or other sacroiliac joint, then the cause of pain probably lies within that joint. If he points over the sciatic trunk in the back of the thigh, very probably he has pathology of neurological origin.

Lower Extremities. In any back problem the legs and the feet may have an important etiological bearing, and they should always be examined. The type of shoes normally worn by the patient should be noted. Of special importance is the sufficiency of the Achilles tendons, or their relative insufficiency. The presence of a marked forefoot drop when the foot is at rest suggests tendo Achillis insufficiency. Unless this tendon is resilient, the heel cannot touch the ground at the same time as the ball of the foot without abnormally stretching the muscles, nerves and blood vessels in the back of the leg. This, in turn, produces abnormal tension on the back muscles and abnormal weight-bearing stresses on all the joints of the foot, leg and back.

Thus, an uncompensated tendo Achillis insufficiency tends to produce knee and hip extension and a flattening of the lumbar lordosis. Overcompensation (i.e., the wearing of high heels dictated by women's fashions) does the reverse, and these people stand with their knees and hips flexed, their lumbar lordosis accentuated, their thoracic kyphosis exaggerated, their cervical lordosis increased, and their heads thrust forward, which materially alters their center of gravity. This disturbs their balance and prevents the maintenance of normal tonus in their supporting muscles. This abnormal posture produces unfair wear and tear in their every joint, from the occiput to those of the toe digits. Muscle pain is their usual complaint, because of constant muscle spasm and fatigue. Joint dysfunction quickly ensues. Such

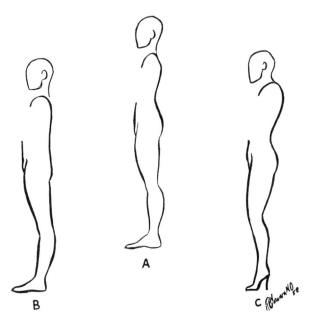

FIGURE 13. (A) Normal posture and normal spinal curves with normally resilient Achilles tendons. (B) The effect of tendo Achillis insufficiency — extension of the knees and hips and flattening of the normal spinal curves. (C) The effect of wearing too high heels — flexion of the knees and hips and accentuation of all the spinal curves.

posture predisposes to acute symptoms whenever minor trauma is inflicted on the joints. Figure 13 illustrates the stress effects which arise from deviations from normal in the Achilles tendons.

Two things must be remembered in adapting shoes to compensate for tendo Achillis insufficiency: (1) correction of the full heel height must never be attempted or whatever resilience is left in the tendon will then be lost; and (2) store shoes can have only a maximum of half an inch added to their heels without producing foot symptoms from the alteration of the slope of the soles of the shoes.

Joint-play Movement

The movements of joint play in the interlaminar joints at each intervertebral junction and at the costovertebral joints, with which we are concerned in the search for dysfunction (which will indicate the level of pathology in the spine), are easy to elicit even though the examining movements used may, at first sight, seem complicated and somewhat nonspecific.

Each movement of joint play at each joint only involves the facets in a range of movement of about ⅛ inch. Yet to achieve this, the part of the back being examined has to be moved through a very wide range of gross movement.

In the normal subject, each movement of joint play can only be elicited at the extreme of some movement within the voluntary range through which that part of the back under review has to be put by the examiner without voluntary muscle assistance by the subject, i.e., passively. When restoring a lost movement of joint play in the patient, the therapeutic manipulative thrust is imparted at the point where the limitation of movement begins.

For instance, in the low back, to elicit the joint-play movement of side tilting at the lumbosacral facet joint on the left, with the patient lying supine, the lumbar spine must first be flattened by flexing the hips and knees to right angles and then the pelvis must be carried to its limit of side bending to the right. These preparatory movements take up all the slack of movement in the area. Then, finally, the pelvis is tilted through an additional few degrees and this opens up the facet joint on the left by about ⅛ inch.

Similarly, to achieve the joint-play movement of side tilt, say at the sixth cervical junction facet joint on the left, the neck has to be carried through its full voluntary range of side bending to the right at this level. Then the index finger of the examining hand is thrust against the fifth cervical vertebra from the right side and this tilts open the facet joint on the left. The total opening movement is probably less than ⅛ inch in extent.

In the same way, to obtain the joint-play movement of, for instance, forward tilting of the facet joints between the fourth and fifth thoracic vertebrae, using the knee-in-the-back method, the thoracic spine above the fifth vertebra must be extended through its full voluntary range; there it is stabilized while the subject is lifted by the examiner, thereby exerting long-axis extension; then the knee thrusts forward against the fifth thoracic vertebra, tilting it backward and opening up the facet joints superiorly between it and the fourth thoracic vertebra. The opening tilt movement again is no greater than ⅛ inch.

It is only possible to stabilize an intervertebral junction so that the specific joint-play movements of its joints can be elicited by taking up all the slack movement, which in the back means putting that area of the back through the voluntary range which is possible at the level being examined.

While the examination techniques are designed to show the range of joint-play movements which is present and normal in health, it is, of course, the deviations from normal which are the signs of disease. These examining movements can all be carried out in patients whose complaints are chronic. It may not be possible to achieve them all in the examination of patients with acute complaints; nevertheless, considerable movement is possible under these circumstances if everything that is done is carried out with great patience and absolute gentleness and if the patient is absolutely supported. *Each movement must be stopped immediately if the patient feels pain.* This is why it is of the greatest importance that these examining techniques should be practiced first on normal subjects. From the normal subject it is safe to progress to the patient with chronic pain. Only when the chronic case can be examined with facility should the acute case be undertaken. It may surprise some how completely the examination can be conducted in an acute case, once the examiner has achieved confidence by learning the techniques exactly.

5

The Low Back

There are twelve interlaminar synovial joints and two sacro-iliac synovial joints which must be examined for joint play in the low back. This includes the joints at the thoracolumbar junction but not the coccygeal joints. There are six intervertebral discs in this area.

The range of joint play at the interlaminar joints consists of long-axis extension, side tilting, and backward tilting. The range of joint play in the sacroiliac joints is a forward and backward torsion movement dissociated from any movement in the sacro-iliac joint of the opposite side.

The patient is examined standing, sitting, supine, in the left and right side-lying positions and prone.

Standing

The patient stands with his back to the examiner and his feet together. He is asked to put one finger over the place that he considers to be the seat of his pain. This localization directs attention to the probable anatomical location of his pathology.

The spine is examined for any general deviation of the curves from normal and any local segmental alteration. The usual segmental change which occurs is either a flattening or reversal of the curves or localized scoliosis.

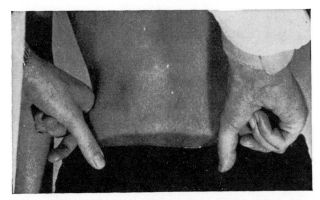

FIGURE 14. Method used to assess the relative heights of the iliac crests with the patient standing.

The relative height of the iliac crests is noted by laying the index fingers over them, keeping the fingers parallel with the floor as illustrated in Figure 14.

If the patient's iliac crest is raised on the side of his pain (particularly if he has indicated the seat of his pain is in relation to the posterior superior iliac spine) and if the convexity of the sciatic scoliosis is toward the same side, the commonly expected pathology is that of sacroiliac joint subluxation or lumbosacral facet joint dysfunction (or both) on that side.

If the iliac crest is raised on the side opposite the seat of pain and the concavity of the scoliosis is on the side of the pain, the common suspected pathology is disc prolapse.

The spine is now palpated, using the three middle fingers of the right hand. The middle finger is placed over the spinous process, and the index and ring fingers respectively in the right and left paraspinal troughs supporting it. The middle finger may detect a minimal vertebral rotation which it might miss if it is used alone because of the ease with which it rolls off the spinous processes.

If during this examination an interspinous step is discovered, this is characteristic of spondylolisthesis. An interspinous dip may be associated with a ruptured interspinous ligament.

Temperature changes of the skin should be noted and any sweat level change may be detected. Skin pigmentation or discoloration is of diagnostic value. Localized swelling should be palpated and its nature assessed.

The patient is now asked to bend forward from the hips, keeping the feet together and the knees straight. The ability to touch the toes is no criterion of normality. The patient should be asked to assess his normal degree of forward bending and any limitation should be determined from this. In forward bending the whole spine should unfold in a smooth synchronous manner, and at the completion of the movement each spinous

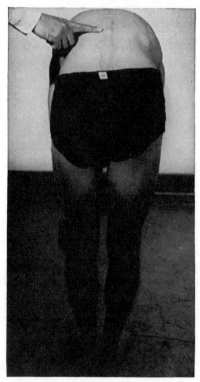

FIGURE 15. Forward-bending position. The spinous processes can clearly be seen and identified.

process should stand out quite distinctly, as illustrated in Figure 15.

At the limit of forward bending percussion over each individual vertebra should be carried out, hitting the vertebra firmly and sharply with the ulnar aspect of the closed fist. Percussion should be done also over the sacroiliac joints.

The patient is then asked to resume the upright position and the spine should fold up in the same smooth synchronous manner as it unfolded.

In a condition which we call "flat back strain" (see page 134) there are two characteristic points which will suggest the diagnosis. First, the patient stoops forward with ease but complains of difficulty in regaining the upright position; second, the symptoms of which he complains had their onset following deep anesthesia, usually administered for some abdominal surgery. Examination of the patient, beyond revealing this difficulty of regaining the upright position, also reveals a flattened lumbar lordosis which the patient cannot arch into its normal curve. There are also signs of dysfunction, often at more than one level in the lumbar spine, and there is abnormal movement at the intervertebral level above the highest level at which dysfunction is demonstrated.

The apparent loss of movement in the lumbar spine, which is sometimes very marked, must not be confused with the loss of movement, which is often very similar, in early cases of ankylosing spondylitis.

These are the only voluntary movements which are used in this clinical examination; all the other examination movements are produced passively by the examiner, as the individual joint movements cannot be elicited in the presence of any voluntary muscle action.

Sitting

The patient now sits on the examining table with his back to the examiner and his lower legs loosely hanging over the edge of the table. The patient should sit equally on both buttocks; the sparing of one buttock may be a valuable clinical sign. The curves of the spine are checked once again. Many people when sitting slouch and their lumbar spines tend to concertina. This is unimportant providing they can resume their normal lordosis painlessly on being asked to sit up.

Upright Rotation. In the upright sitting position the hands are locked behind the neck and the movements of upright rotation to the right (Fig. 16) and to the left are performed.

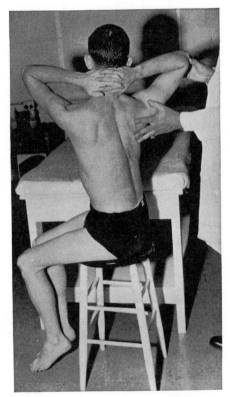

FIGURE 16. Upright rotation in the sitting position. Note the virtual absence of rotation in the lumbar spine and the exaggerated lateral curve in the thoracic spine.

Upright rotation will only be limited by loss of function in the sacroiliac joint on the side to which the patient is turned or by pathology at the lumbosacral junction. Pathology elsewhere in the lumbar spine should not limit upright rotation, because there is virtually no intervertebral rotation in the lumbar spine.

Back Lying with Rotation. The back-lying position is then adopted. The patient flops back on the examiner. The patient's legs should remain relaxed and dangling. Back lying in this manner throws a strain on the lumbosacral junction, and pathology here may limit this part of the examination. Again, passivity on the part of the patient must be stressed. In the back-lying position the trunk is rotated to the right and left. As soon as the ischial tuberosity on the side away from which the trunk is being turned leaves the couch, a marked backward torsion strain is exerted on the sacroiliac joint on the side toward which rotation is directed. If this position is now maintained, and if pressure is exerted by the examiner's free hand vertically over the anterior superior spine on the side on which the ischial

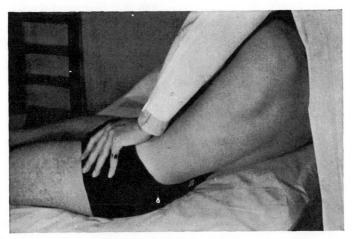

FIGURE 17. Examining movement of back lying with rotation to the right and exertion of backward torsion on the left sacroiliac joint. The patient is in the sitting position.

tuberosity is raised from the couch, a marked backward torsion strain is put on the sacroiliac joint of this side; this action will relieve the backward torsion strain on the other sacroiliac joint and may indeed produce a mild forward torsion strain on it. Put another way, back lying with rotation of the trunk to the right exerts a marked backward torsion on the right sacroiliac joint which is relieved by backward torsion exerted through the left sacroiliac joint. Figure 17 demonstrates this rather complicated maneuver.

Measurements. Finally, in the sitting position, the distance between the posterior superior iliac spines is measured. This measurement should be compared with the distance between these bony points when the patient eventually assumes the prone position.

It is my clinical observation that normally there is an increase in the distance between the posterior superior iliac spines of from ¼ to ¾ inch when measured sitting and then lying prone. In the absence of this change of distance with change of posture there is sacroiliac joint disease. This is perhaps the earliest sign of ankylosing spondylitis. This movement between the iliac bones with change of posture is surely the best proof, if proof be needed, of movement in the sacroiliac joints in a normal person.

Supine

The patient then lies on his back. In this position leg measurements are made and a neurological examination of the legs is undertaken.

Measurements. Muscle group atrophy is detected by measuring the circumference of the thighs and calves at points 6 inches above and 6 inches below the patella.

To use anything but a ½-inch cloth tape is courting error. A metal tape cannot assume the contours of the leg. A thin pocket tape is easily placed around the leg obliquely without the obliquity being noticed; it can also be pulled and, unnoticed, indent the soft tissues to varying degrees. When measuring the thigh, the patella must be pushed down to the limit of its caudal movement so that it becomes a fixed bony point from which to measure. When measuring the calf, the patella must be pushed up to the limit of its cephalad range so that again it becomes a fixed bony point from which to measure. The distance of 6 inches from the patella is chosen to avoid errors from atrophy of the vastus medialis or swelling in the suprapatellar pouch, both of which may be due to knee joint pathology.

The true leg lengths are then measured from beneath the anterior superior iliac spines to below the medial tibial malleoli. In performing these measurements the markings on the tape are ignored at first. The length of the tape is transferred from one leg to the other, and any difference in the length of the longer leg can be accurately read off by sliding the thumb at the foot end down the tape until it comes to rest below the malleolus.

Less than ½-inch discrepancy in these measurements may usually be ignored as being due to human error. However, it should always be noted and on occasion may be of significance. A short leg seldom if ever causes back pain, but it may maintain back pain or provoke a recurrence of back pain. In the average back problem, the equalizing of leg lengths is not, by itself, a treatment for pain.

The feet should then be examined with particular attention being paid to the resiliency of the Achilles tendons. Figures 18 and 19 show the method used to determine the optimum height of heel which the patient requires to compensate for any tendo Achillis insufficiency. A duralumin strip is shaped to the contour of the inner border of the foot at rest (Fig. 18). This contoured strip is then removed from the foot and put on a

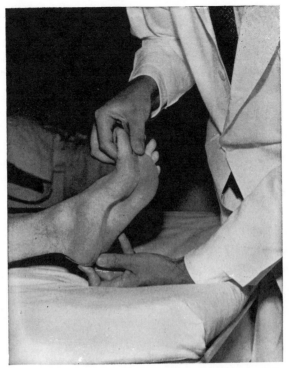

FIGURE 18.   Method used to assess the contour of the foot at rest, the prerequisite of determining the heel height required to compensate for tendo Achillis insufficiency.

firm table. A book is placed under the heel part of the metal strip and leafed open until the flat heel part of the strip is parallel to the floor (Fig. 19). This height is measured and is the height of heel required to correct the weight bearing of all the weight-bearing joints. But it will be recalled (page 53) that raising the heels of shoes to the full height is not recommended.

Neurological Examination. The four leg reflexes are elicited, namely, the cremasteric (labial) reflex, whose reflex arc is at the level of the first and second lumbar nerves; the patellar tendon reflex, whose arc is at the level of the third and fourth lumbar

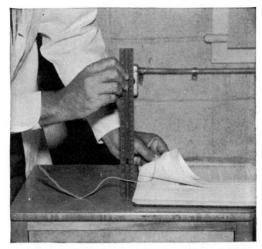

FIGURE 19. The duralumin strip is removed from the foot and the heel part of the contour is supported on an open book. The correct heel height is measured when the flat part of the heel contour is parallel to the table top.

nerves; the tendo Achillis reflex, whose arc is at the level of the first and second sacral nerves; and the plantar reflex, anomalies of which indicate pyramidal tract pathology. It should be remembered that there is an overlap in level of these reflex arcs and their changes do not necessarily accurately localize a level of pathology.

Sensory changes are now looked for. For our purposes, eliciting sensation to pin prick is sufficient, though in confusing cases light touch, vibration, position, and deep sensation (by pinching the Achilles tendons) may have to be tested. Sensory dermatomes are seldom accurate in determining levels of pathology in back conditions, but the mere presence of sensory changes is important. The main thing is to remember to prick the same area on each leg front and back. The anal reflex will be elicited in pricking in the saddle area. This reflex has its arc at the fourth and fifth sacral levels.

The reflexes mentioned are the common ones elicited, but it will be noted that there remains a gap in the cord levels through which the reflex arcs pass, namely, the fifth lumbar level, and a hamstring reflex can be elicited to cover this level.

> All these reflexes are concerned with striated voluntary muscles, having their centers within the cerebrospinal axis, and may be inhibited by voluntary effort. Further, following spine surgery there may be a neurological deficit unconnected with the current problem, so not too much reliance can be placed on doubtful neurological signs. However, a useful clinical observation is that the absence of one cremasteric reflex may be the only early physical sign of a neurogenic tumor.

The next step is to rule out the presence of hip joint pathology, so that signs from the hip will not be confused with other signs when moving the hip during examination. This is conveniently done by rolling the outstretched leg inward and outward, these being the only hip movements which can be performed without moving other joints as well.

Straight-leg-raising Test. The straight-leg-raising test is without doubt one of the most erroneously performed and the most poorly interpreted tests in common use. Limitation of straight-leg-raising by pain either in the low back or the back of the leg or both is not specifically indicative of radiculitis.

Straight-leg-raising may be limited and painful because of any of three conditions: (1) tight hamstring muscles; (2) sacroiliac joint pathology; and (3) radiculitis. Any of these conditions limits unilateral straight-leg-raising by pain of sciatic distribution. Tightness of the hamstrings can be determined by palpation, and pain from this is usually, but not always, felt behind the knee. This should have been assessed while the patient was examined standing and stooping, but it can be checked again now. It is not a sign of normality to be able to raise the straight leg to 90 degrees. It is usually abnormal to go beyond this angle. Having assessed hamstring muscle tightness, it remains to differentiate between sacroiliac joint pathology and radiculitis.

At a certain angle of straight-leg-raising the hamstrings pull on their origin at the ischial tuberosity, and because the opposite leg is stabilizing the other half of the pelvis, the os innominatum on the side being tested tends to be rotated backward on the sacrum through the sacroiliac joint when this muscle pull increases. At about the same angle tension is being put on the sciatic nerve roots through pull on the sciatic trunk. Pathology in the sacroiliac joint or radiculitis produces pain either in the low back, buttock or back of the leg. If the leg is then dropped ½ to 1 inch, both the stress on the joint and the pull on the nerve roots are relieved. Then with the leg stationary, the foot is dorsiflexed. No painful stress is added to the sacroiliac joint, but a pull is reinstituted on the nerve roots through the nerve trunk. Exacerbation of pain on dorsiflexion of the foot is the true Lasègue sign of radiculitis. If the pain is not reproduced by dorsiflexing the foot, sacroiliac joint pathology should be suspected.

A doubtful Lasègue sign can be checked by using Naffziger's bilateral jugular vein compression test. This test increases the pressure of the spinal fluid, which in turn increases the pressure effect of a tumor in the epidural space. It may also be checked by the head-leg test in which tension is exerted on the low spinal roots by pulling upon them from the head end.

Both legs are now raised together, keeping the knees extended. In this movement the hamstring muscles pull equally at their origins on both sides, tilting the pelvis backward as a whole at the lumbosacral junction. This tilting tends to occur at an earlier angle of elevation than that at which sacroiliac joint movement takes place; hence, pain at an earlier angle with both legs raised together than with either raised by itself almost certainly indicates lumbosacral joint dysfunction.

Side Bending of the Pelvis. The knees and hips are now flexed, with the forelegs dropping over the examiner's forearm and the hips being kept at 90 degrees. In this position the lumbar spine is flattened and its interlaminar joints tend to be locked except at the lumbosacral junction. When the pelvis is bent to the right (Fig. 20), the lumbosacral facet joint on the left is opened. The lumbosacral intervertebral disc tends to be compressed on the right. Conversely, if the pelvis is bent to the left, the lumbosacral interlaminar joint is opened on the right and the disc tends to be compressed on the left.

> Limitation of side bending of the pelvis both to the right and left by pain indicated as being at the lumbosacral junction suggests disc pathology or bone disease.

Figure 20 illustrates the movement of side bending of the pelvis to the right. Some vertical downward pressure has to be put on the femoral shafts to maintain the locking of the rest of the lumbar spinal joints and to control the movement. Side tilting at the higher facet joints in the lumbar spine can be elicited at the limit of side bending of the pelvis while lifting the sacrum from the couch. The lift is made a little higher as each higher level is examined. This technique is most accurate for examining the lumbosacral junction.

To complete the examination of the patient in the supine position the leg pulses must be examined, as Leriche's syndrome may mimic low back pathology. Also the abdominal examination should be performed at this time.

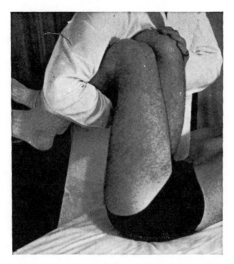

FIGURE 20.   Side bending of the pelvis to the right to open up the interlaminar articulations on the left. The lumbar spine is flattened by flexion
of the hips.

Side-lying Positions

The side-lying position is then adopted by the patient, first
on one side and then on the other. The following examining
movements are carried out on each side.

Left Side Lying. The first part of this examination is directed
at further differentiation between sacroiliac joint and lumbosacral junction pathology. This is sometimes very necessary
when signs up to this point have been unclear. In a circular
area less than 3 inches in diameter, whose center is the posterior
superior iliac spine, there are five anatomical centers in which
commonly there may be pathology and from which almost
identical symptoms of low back pain radiating down the back
of the leg may arise. The reader is referred to page 77 for
details.

With the patient in the left side-lying position, the left leg is drawn up onto the chest and held there by the patient. The examiner then extends the right leg, supporting the lower leg, with the knee flexed at right angles. This static position (Fig. 21) is maintained for a short time and then the left leg is released (Fig. 22), while extension on the right leg is maintained.

Pain in this static position felt on the left suggests sacroiliac joint dysfunction; this pain should be relieved immediately when the patient releases the left leg. The backward torsion strain on the sacroiliac joint which is exerted by the fully flexed left leg pulling against the stress of the extended right leg is relieved by release of the left leg. If, however, the static position is painless but pain is experienced on release of the left leg then lumbosacral junction pathology should be suspected. This is because on release of the left leg the tension exerted by the examiner on the extended right leg causes a quick tilt of the pelvis on the fifth lumbar vertebra.

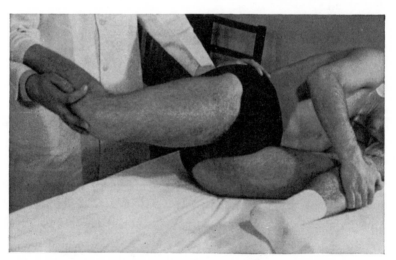

FIGURE 21. The static position adopted in differentiating between sacro-iliac and lumbosacral junction pain. In the left side-lying position the joints on the left are considered.

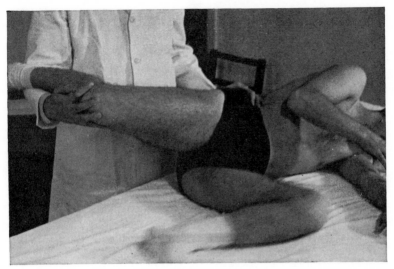

FIGURE 22. Release of the left leg from the static position illustrated in Figure 21. The upper part of the right leg is not moved during this examining movement.

Iliotibial Band Resiliency. The left leg when released falls naturally into a flexed position of 90 degrees at the hip and 90 degrees at the knee, and the patient is asked to hold the knee down on the couch in this position. Meanwhile the examiner lets his holding hand slide down to the ankle. The right leg is then further abducted and extended so that the iliotibial band lies over the greater trochanter of the femur (Fig. 23). The elevating hold of the right leg is then relaxed so that the knee may drop to the table. When the iliotibial band is pathologically tight, the knee remains suspended. When it is normally resilient, the knee falls readily to the table top. Usually there is diffuse fibrositic tenderness in a tight iliotibial band.

The role of the iliotibial band in back pain is not sufficiently recognized. Its significance is discussed in Chapter 10, page 154.

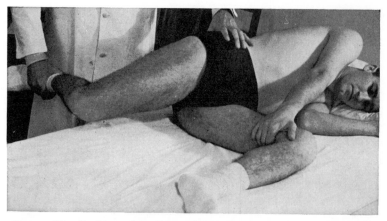

FIGURE 23. Position adopted in performing Ober's test for tightness in the right iliotibial band. The right knee should drop to the couch without trouble.

Forward Torsion. The position of the patient's legs is then reversed, the right leg dropping in front of the lower left leg. The patient's trunk is rotated backward until all the intervertebral spinal movement is achieved, and the interlaminar joints are

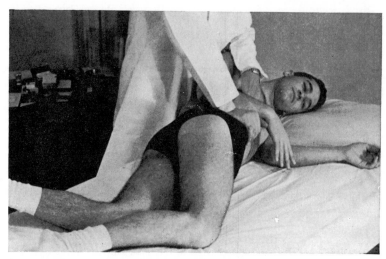

FIGURE 24. Position adopted for performing the forward-torsion examination of the right sacroiliac joint.

locked by pulling on the right shoulder and upper lateral aspect of the trunk by the examiner's left elbow and forearm. His right hand holds the patient's right wrist. The reason for this is that if the wrist is not relaxed the back is not, and the next examining movement of forward torsion on the right sacroiliac joint cannot be performed. This movement is achieved by exerting a downward and somewhat oblique thrust directed caudally over the anterior third of the patient's iliac crest, using the thenar eminence of the hand. Figure 24 illustrates this maneuver.

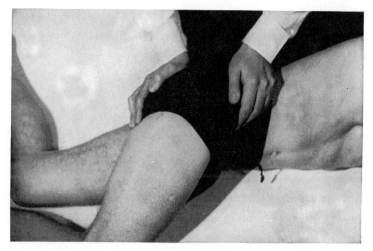

FIGURE 25. Position adopted for performing the backward-torsion examination of the right sacroiliac joint in the left side-lying position.

Backward Torsion. Backward torsion on the right sacroiliac joint is again produced (see Fig. 17) by pulling backward on the patient's anterior superior iliac spine with the left hand and pushing forward over the ischial tuberosity with the right hand. Figure 25 illustrates this examining movement.

Right Side Lying. The patient then assumes the right side-lying position and the examining movements which have been described in the left side-lying position are repeated — namely, backward torsion on the right sacroiliac joint, movement at the lumbosacral junction, the left iliotibial band resiliency, and forward and backward torsion on the left sacroiliac joint. The details of examination in this position will not be described as they are identical with those above.

Prone

The patient now assumes the face-down or prone position. The distance between the posterior superior iliac spines is measured for the second time and comparison made of this measurement with that noted when the patient was in the upright sitting position. In the absence of sacroiliac joint disease there should be a spread of these spines of up to ¾ inch.

Skin Rolling. The next examining procedure is that of skin rolling up the spine. This is both difficult to describe and to illustrate. It is a smooth rolling of the skin over the spinous processes of the vertebrae by the forefingers over the advancing thumbs. Figure 26 shows how the skin is picked up preparatory to rolling it. Skin rolling is then performed over each side of the back, and fibrositic infiltration and trigger pain points are demonstrated by tightness and acute tenderness.

It is my clinical observation that there will be tightness and tenderness, maximum over the level of bone pathology or over the vertebra above the level of joint or disc pathology.

Direct Vertical Thrust. The level of probable bone, joint or disc pathology as determined by the skin rolling test is confirmed by the next examining movement, namely, a direct vertical thrust over each individual vertebra. To avoid an abnormal rotatory movement during this movement, the thrust is achieved by flex-

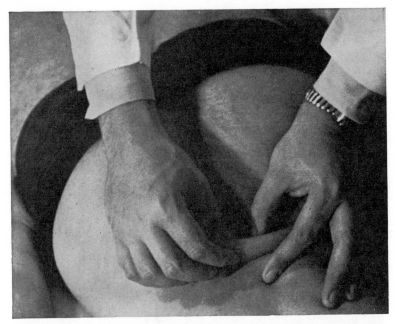

FIGURE 26. Manner in which the skin is picked up between the thumbs and index fingers to perform the maneuver of skin rolling.

ing the forefinger to place the horizontal middle phalanx on one side of the spinous process and the hyperextended terminal phalanx of the thumb on the other side of the spinous process (Fig. 27). This cradles the spinous process between the thumb and forefinger and the downward thrust is equal over the lateral masses on each side. This movement is performed over each lumbar vertebra.

Should there still be some doubt as to level of pathology it can be checked further by extending (NOT hyperextending) the lumbar spine by lifting the legs, and with the back stationary exerting a downward thrust with the thenar eminence of the other hand over each vertebra. Figure 28 illustrates this maneuver.

These last two thrusting movements elicit the normal joint-play movement of backward tilting of the interlaminar facet

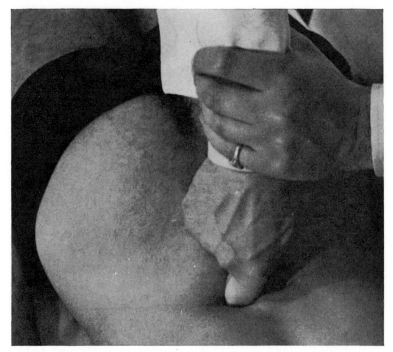

FIGURE 27.   Direct pressure over a specific vertebra. The spinous process
is cradled between the thumb and the flexed index finger to avoid unnatural rotation of the vertebra during the thrusting movement.

joints. A therapeutic manipulative movement which may be used
to restore this is described later (see pages 123–124 and Figs. 57
and 58).

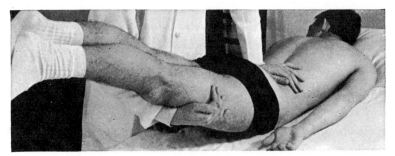

FIGURE 28.   Method used to exert direct pressure over a specific vertebra, using as a counter force extension of the lumbar spine.

Palpation. Finally there are fourteen local areas in which tenderness on palpation is very constant in certain conditions. There are five areas on each side of the back to be examined and one in each buttock and one in the back of each thigh. The back areas are illustrated in Figure 29A and the underlying anatomy is demonstrated in Figure 29B.

(1) One finger breadth medial to the posterior superior iliac spine is the most superficial posterior ligament of the sacroiliac joint. Tenderness here suggests sacroiliac joint pathology.

(2) One finger breadth lateral to the posterior superior iliac spine is the puny part of the gluteal muscle origin which may be torn by minor trauma. Tenderness here suggests the pathology of a muscle tear.

(3) One finger breadth above the posterior superior iliac spine is where the sacrospinalis muscle joins its tendon. Muscle fiber tears frequently occur at this junction with minor lifting trauma. Tenderness here suggests this pathology.

(4) One finger breadth above and medial to the posterior superior iliac spine is the area over the interlaminar facet joint, where tenderness may be felt if dysfunction is present.

(5) One finger breadth medial and inferior to (4) is the area where local tenderness may be felt from disc pathology.

(6) Tenderness lateral to the ischial tuberosity where the sciatic trunk emerges from beneath the pyriformis muscle suggests either tightness of the muscle or radicular pathology.

(7) Tenderness on rolling with the fingers deeply over the sciatic trunk in the back of the thigh indicates neuritis.

Rectal and Pelvic Examination. The low back examination is then completed by doing a rectal and, if necessary, a pelvic examination. The lower ligaments of the sacroiliac joints can be palpated and in some people the anterior aspect of the lumbo-

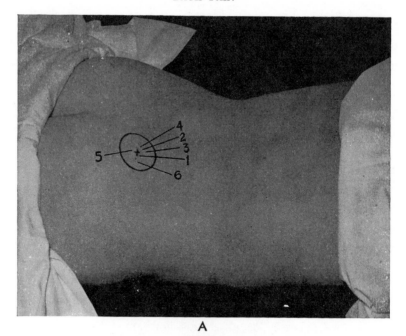

A

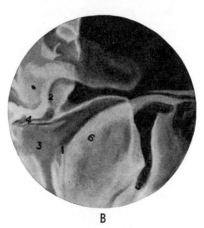

B

FIGURE 29. Anatomical seats of pathology which can give rise to pain in the low back radiating down the leg. (A) Circular area of about 1½-inch radius with center at posterior superior iliac spine; (B) drawing of an X-ray picture of same area shown in (A). (1) Posterior superior iliac spine; (2) lumbosacral apophyseal joint pathology; (3) sacrospinalis tear; (4) disc pathology; (5) sacroiliac joint pathology; (6) gluteal origin tear.

sacral junction can be felt. The whole of the sacrum should be palpated anteriorly.

Coccygeal Joints. The opportunity is taken, at this time, to examine the coccygeal joints in which the movement of joint play is an anteroposterior tilt, using the finger within the rectum and the thumb externally alternately as pivot and pusher.

6

The Thoracic Spine

There are twenty-four interlaminar synovial joints, including those at the cervicothoracic junction but not those at the thoraco-lumbar junction, and at each level (except the first, eleventh and twelfth ribs, where there are only two) four costovertebral joints and two costotransverse joints, making eighty-four in all. As it is not possible clinically to differentiate between these small rib articulations, each group of three is considered together. For practical purposes, then, the total number of synovial joints to be examined for joint play in this part of the spine is forty-eight. There are twelve intervertebral discs in this area.

The movements of joint play at the interlaminar joints are (1) long axis-extension, (2) rotation, (3) backward tilting.

The patient is examined standing, sitting, prone, and in the left and right side-lying position.

Standing

The patient is asked to indicate the seat of the pain.

The line of the spinous processes is palpated from the seventh cervical vertebra downward, using the middle finger of the right hand supported by the index finger and the ring finger in the paravertebral troughs. The three fingers are run smoothly down the spine without stopping to feel each individual process but rather to note segmental deviation from the midline which may not be appreciated by gross inspection alone. The shawl areas of the trapezii muscles are palpated by picking them up between the thumb and fingers and feeling for any spasm or tender spots.

The patient is asked to bend forward and the synchronous spreading of the spinous processes is observed. In this position each vertebra is percussed serially, and any localized pain is assessed. The patient is then asked to assume the upright standing position and the synchronous manner in which the spinous processes resume their normal relationship is observed. The respiratory excursion is then measured.

Sitting

The patient then sits on the examining couch with his legs dangling freely over the edge and with the fingers locked behind the neck. He is turned to the right and the left and limitation

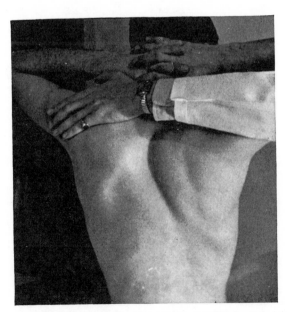

FIGURE 30. Examining position for upright rotation to the right in the sitting position.

of motion is noted, limitation of motion in either direction indi-
cating dysfunction on that side (Fig. 30).

Joint Play of First and Second Costovertebral Joints. While the
patient is in the sitting position, the joint play of the first and
second costovertebral joints is examined. To examine these joints
on the right side, the patient grasps the left shoulder with the
right hand and places the left hand on the right forearm near
the elbow, pulling the right shoulder anteriorly and medially.
The examiner places the ulnar border of his right fist at the base
of the neck on the right, grasps his right wrist with his left hand
and pushes the head forward and to the left with his left forearm,
thereby exposing the angle of the first rib. Figure 31 demon-

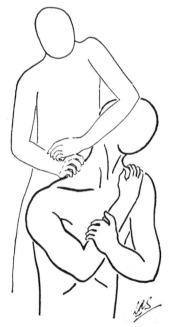

FIGURE 31. Position adopted for examination of the normal range of
joint play in the costovertebral joints of the first and second ribs, the
patient being in the sitting position.

strates the position. The patient is then asked to exhale completely and, at the beginning of inspiration, a downward springing thrust is made by both hands over the angle of the rib. This opens up the costovertebral articulations, separating the articulations of the rib from those of the transverse process and the two articular surfaces on the adjacent vertebral bodies.

The costovertebral articulations of the second rib are next examined. In this case the patient pulls the shoulder around further and the examiner pushes the head further forward and laterally (see Fig. 31). The right fist is moved slightly backward and laterally to rest on the angle of the second rib. At the beginning of inspiration the springing thrust is again applied. The left side is examined in an analogous manner.

Prone

Skin Rolling. The patient then adopts the prone position with the hands under his chest. Skin rolling is performed over the thoracic spine from below upward, the skin being picked up between the thumbs and forefingers. As the thumbs are pushed up toward the head, the skin is rolled backward over them by the forefingers. Tightness and tenderness at any level indicates pathology in the bone or joints at that level. Skin rolling is then performed over the paravertebral areas to detect localized fibrositic infiltration or areas of muscle pathology.

Direct Vertical Thrust. A nonspecific examining movement of the interlaminar facet joints and discs at each level is obtained by springing each vertebra forward. To do this the spinous process is cradled between the end of the thumb and middle phalanx of the flexed forefinger (Fig. 32). The thumb and finger thrust forward and superiorly equally on either side over the

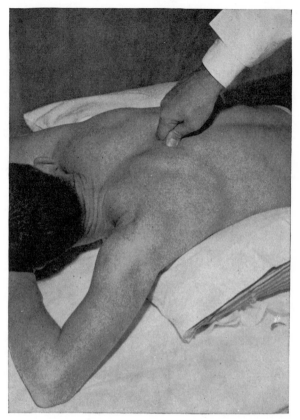

FIGURE 32.   Direct thrust over the sixth thoracic vertebra. Pain elicited
by direct pressure in this manner suggests pathology at the junction below
the vertebra or pathology in the vertebra.

transverse processes. This avoids any rotation of the vertebra.
Pressure downward is applied to take up the slack, and then an
additional springing thrust is applied in the same direction. Any
discomfort on the part of the patient is noted and indicates
pathology in the joints or discs between this vertebra and the
one immediately below it. The process is started at the twelfth
thoracic vertebra and carried upward to the seventh cervical
vertebra.

Backward Tilt. The backward tilt of each pair of inter-laminar joints is checked by stabilizing the vertebra above the level of the joints being examined and applying a thrust on the dorsal process of the vertebra below the joints. This is done with the patient lying on his crossed forearms. The examiner places his left forearm beneath those of the patient and lifts away from the table to take up slack. Then pressure is applied through the ulnar aspect of his right hand. Figure 33 demon-strates the position adopted in applying pressure over the eighth thoracic vertebra.

A sharp springing motion, which is toward the table and inferiorly, slides the vertebra forward and caudally and opens the interlaminar facet joints between the sprung vertebra and the one above it. The examining process is then carried stepwise

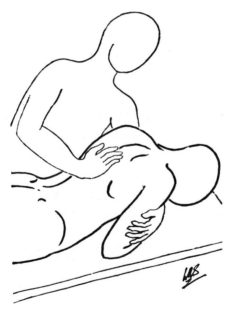

FIGURE 33. One method of producing the movement of joint play, open-ing up the superior aspect of an interlaminar intervertebral joint at one level.

down the vertebrae. At each lower level the patient's chest must be lifted further from the table to take up the additional slack.

Interlaminar Joint Rotation. In this movement each thoracic vertebra is rotated on the one directly below it to produce the movement of rotation in the range of joint play. This movement is necessary before painless voluntary movement of rotation of the thoracic spine as a whole can take place. Examination is necessary to determine if one or more of these facet joints are locked in partial rotation.

The patient drops his right arm over the edge of the couch. The examiner places his left forearm beneath the shoulder in front of the axilla to raise the chest wall from the couch, taking up the slack of voluntary rotation above this level. At this point the examiner places the ulnar edge of his right hand to the right of the spinous process of the fourth thoracic vertebra, which places it over the right transverse process of this vertebra. A sharp thrust downward, into the couch, and slightly toward the feet is made, producing the movement of joint play of rotation to the right at this level. The third thoracic vertebra and those above it have been stabilized by the rotation of that upper part of the spine during the movement of raising the chest wall from the couch. Figure 34 illustrates this maneuver.

The shoulder is then raised a short distance further from the couch, taking up the additional slack of normal movement between the fourth and fifth thoracic vertebrae, so that the joint play between the fifth and sixth thoracic vertebrae may now be examined in the same way. This examining process is continued down the thoracic spine to the twelfth vertebra. The examiner then moves to the other side of the couch; the patient drops the left arm over the edge of the couch and the left side of the chest is raised. Then the joint-play rotation to the left of the interlaminar joints of the thoracic spine is examined.

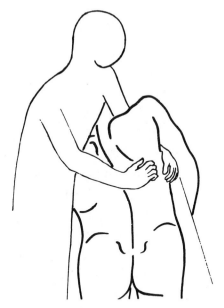

FIGURE 34.   Position adopted when performing the examination to elicit
rotation to the right of a thoracic vertebra.

Side-lying Positions

Left Side Lying. The patient is now asked to lie on his left side.
The upper leg rests in front of the lower leg on the couch; the
back is vertical to the table; the right arm lies loosely across the
chest.

Springing of the Ribs. In the following maneuvers the costovertebral joint-play movements are examined at the rib junctions,
from the third to the twelfth ribs.

Ribs three through six must be sprung through the vertebral
border of the scapula. The position of examination is illustrated
in Figure 35. The patient's right shoulder is grasped by the
examiner's left hand. The third finger rests in the anterior axillary
fold and the palm of the hand rests over the acromion process.
This hand pulls and rotates the shoulder girdle and scapula

backward toward the spine and stabilizes it in this position. The
ulnar border of the right hand is placed over the scapula at
the angle of the third rib and a sharp springing thrust is made
anteriorly, inferiorly, and slightly laterally. During the thrust
the hand turns in a counterclockwise rotation. The purpose of
this movement is to pull the rib away from its vertebral and
transverse process articulations. As the thrust is made, the
patient's shoulder is pulled slightly backward at the same time.
This maneuver is necessarily complicated because of the spatial
relationship of the rib articulations which are to be moved. If
the relation of the head of the rib to the vertebral column is
remembered, and if it is realized that it is necessary to separate
these two bones at three articulations to produce the movement
of joint play, the reader may come to an understanding of the

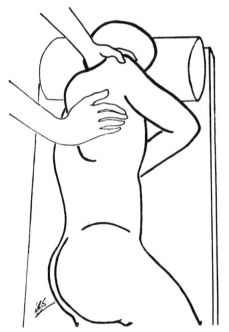

FIGURE 35.   Position adopted in examining for the normal range of
joint play in the costovertebral joints from the third to the sixth rib.

movement which is necessary. The thrust is made at the end of full expiration just as inspiration begins. The hand is placed serially over the angles of the fourth, fifth, and sixth ribs as each is examined.

The patient then places the right arm up over the head to grasp the head end of the couch. This swings the scapula anteriorly and away from the angle of the seventh rib and those below it. The examiner no longer holds on to the shoulder, but places the left hand over the right one to direct its movement. The right hand is placed on the angle of the rib and again the rotatory thrusting movement is imparted to the rib. Figure 36 illustrates how the scapula is drawn away, exposing the angles of the lower ribs, and the position adopted to spring them. The ribs on the left are not examined at this point, but this maneuver must later

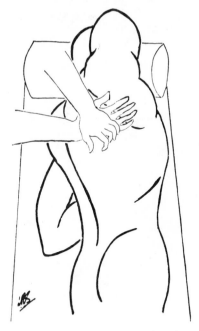

FIGURE 36. Position adopted in examining for the normal range of joint play in the costovertebral joints from the seventh rib downward.

be repeated on the other side with the patient in the right side-lying position.

Rotation of Cervicothoracic Vertebrae. The joint-play rotation of the interlaminar joints between the seventh cervical and the first thoracic, the first and second thoracic, and the second and third and the third and fourth thoracic vertebrae is then examined.

The head is cradled in the examiner's left arm. The tips of the fingers grasp the chin and the left parietal area of the skull rests on the left forearm. The right thumb is placed on the upper lateral aspect of the spinous process of the seventh cervical

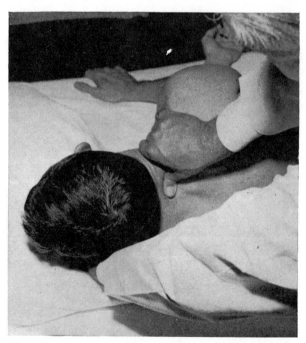

FIGURE 37. Position of the thumb over the lateral aspect of the spinous process of either the seventh cervical or the first, second or third thoracic vertebra to produce the movement of joint play of junction rotation found at these levels. This figure should be studied with Figure 38 which shows the same position from the front.

vertebra; the fingers of the hand rest on the side of the neck which is uppermost. The vertex of the skull is carried upward as the chin is carried downward until the seventh cervical spinous process is felt to begin to move upward against the thumb. At this point the head is stabilized and a springing thrust imparted to the spinous process, producing the movement of rotation in joint play between the seventh cervical and first thoracic vertebrae. Figures 37 and 38 show the examining position from the front and back.

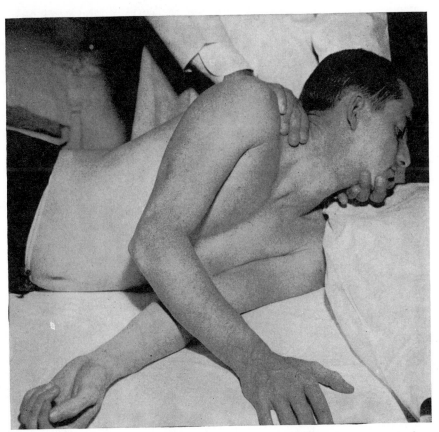

FIGURE 38. Front view of the position adopted to produce the movement of joint play of rotation at the cervicothoracic and upper three interthoracic junctions.

The thumb is then moved over the lateral aspect of the spinous process of the first thoracic vertebra. The head is carried further upward until this spinous process is felt to move. At this point a springing thrust is made on it, producing the rotatory movement of joint play between the first and second thoracic vertebrae. This maneuver is then carried out for the third and fourth thoracic vertebrae.

Right Side Lying. At this point the patient assumes the right side-lying position and the examination of the costovertebral joints and the interlaminar joints of the cervicothoracic region on the left side is made. The techniques are, of course, the same as those described for these joints on the right side in the two preceding paragraphs.

Neurological Examination

The neurological examination of the chest for levels of pathology may help in diagnosis. Sensory levels are segmental and much more accurate than in the limbs. A level at which sweat on the skin changes is also a helpful clinical sign.

> It should be remembered that, for clinical purposes, if the pathology from which the symptoms are emanating is in the thoracic portion of the spinal cord, the level of the pathological lesion is usually two segments higher than the detected sensory or sweat changes.

Both superficial and deep reflex changes may assist in diagnosis, but after the triceps reflex, whose arc is at the first thoracic level, there is a gap until the sixth thoracic level is reached. The epigastric reflex, whose reflex arc is between the sixth and eighth thoracic levels, is elicited by stroking below and along the costal margin, and elicits contraction of the upper fibers of the transversalis muscle with dimpling of the epigastrium on the side being tested. The usual upper quadrant abdominal reflex is controlled through the eighth to tenth thoracic levels and the lower abdominal quadrant reflex through the eleventh and twelfth thoracic levels. To cross check, there are two less specific periosteal reflexes, namely, the costo-abdominal and the pubic reflexes. The costo-abdominal reflex is elicited by tapping the costal margin in the nipple line, resulting in pulling up of the umbilicus on the same side. The arcs of this reflex are the eighth and ninth thoracic levels. The pubic reflex, which is the least specific as its segmental level covers from the sixth to the twelfth thoracic levels, is elicited by tapping the pubis, as a result of which there is a general contraction of the abdominal muscles (but especially the recti) and contraction of the adductors of the thighs.

Palpation

Palpation of the intercostal muscles, the ribs and the costochondral junctions must be done, the sternum, breasts and axillae must be examined and the viscera of the chest and upper abdomen must be assessed before the examination of the thoracic part of the back can be considered complete.

7

The Cervical Spine

There are fourteen synovial interlaminar joints; this does not include the joints at the cervicothoracic junction. There are also twelve joints of Luschka, and the odontoid-atlas joint in this area. Though there is a range of joint play at the odontoid-atlas joint, it cannot be specifically demonstrated by clinical means, nor can individual movement be demonstrated in the joints of Luschka. This leaves fourteen joints to be examined for joint play. There are five intervertebral discs in this area.

The range of movement of joint play at the interlaminar joints is: (1) long-axis extension; (2) anteroposterior glide; (3) side glide; (4) at the occipito-atlanto-axial joints, rotation; and (5) at the joints between the third and seventh cervical junctions, side tilt.

The patient is examined standing and supine. It must be remembered, however, that when a patient who has neck pain is being examined, the left and right side-lying positions and the prone position must also be used to examine the joints of the cervicothoracic junction and the upper four to six thoracic junctions as described in Chapter 6.

Standing

Observe the way the head is held. The patient then indicates the place he considers to be the seat of his pain.

94

It is of clinical significance that if the head is turned away from the side of the pain, the neck is bent toward the side of the pain and the face is tilted upward, the cause of symptoms is usually physical; whereas, if the neck is tilted toward the side of the pain, the head is turned toward the same side and the face is tilted down, the cause is oftentimes hysterical.

The spinous processes of the cervical vertebrae and the upper six thoracic vertebrae are then palpated, using the middle finger supported on each side by the index and ring fingers. Any spasm of the neck muscles is noted. The trapezii are palpated between the thumb and fingers over the shawl area and any spasm or tender spots are noted.

The patient is asked to demonstrate his voluntary range of movement in flexion, extension, rotation and side bending.

Supine

The patient then lies on his back. The voluntary range of motion is now checked by the examiner. In this position it may be noted that the seat of the patient's pain is in fact located in the upper thoracic spine, whereas when the movements were undertaken by use of the voluntary muscles while standing, they appeared to be in the neck. Now the range of movement of joint play is examined.

Long-axis Extension. The chin is dropped onto the neck (Fig. 39) to flatten the cervical lordosis. Figure 40A shows the normal cervical lordosis, and Figure 40B shows the lordosis flattened by dropping the chin. The examiner's left hand is placed under the occiput and his right hand steadies the chin to prevent flexion or extension during the performance of the movement of joint play of long-axis extension. A steady pull is applied chiefly through the left hand on the occiput until the traction overcomes the friction of the patient on the couch and the body starts to move.

If the patient develops muscle spasm and pain later in the examination, repeating this movement will relieve these symptoms.

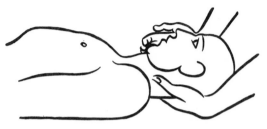

FIGURE 39. Position adopted prior to exerting long-axis traction. The left hand pulls while the right hand steadies the chin, which is dropped down onto the neck to flatten the cervical lordosis.

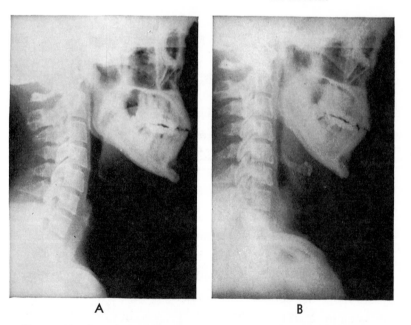

A   B

FIGURE 40. Long-axis extension. (A) Normal cervical lordosis of the spine; (B) cervical lordosis flattened by simply dropping the chin onto the neck. It is only in the flattened position that long-axis extension can be efficiently applied.

Figure 41 illustrates the long-axis extension; the X-ray in Figure 42A shows the vertebrae before traction; the X-ray in Figure 42B shows the effect of long-axis extension.

In this movement the rules of manipulative techniques are

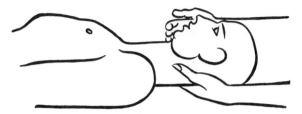

FIGURE 41. Position at the completion of long-axis extension. Note there has been no flexion or extension of the head on the neck. Most of the pull has been exerted from the occiput.

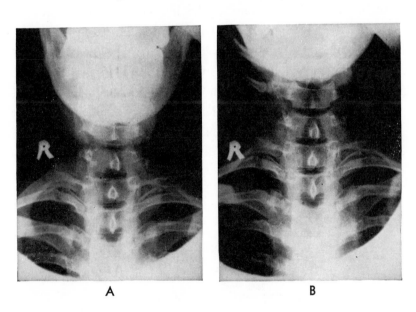

FIGURE 42. Long-axis extension. (A) Cervical spine at rest; (B) cervical spine at the extreme of the movement of long-axis extension. The wide opening of the intervertebral spaces is apparent when compared with their position at rest (A). The mandible is one and a half vertebrae higher up the spine.

deliberately broken in that this movement of joint play is elicited in all the joints of the cervical spine at the same time.

Anteroposterior Glide. To elicit the anterior part of this movement the head and neck are carried forward through their full arc of movement without tilting the head, the face being kept parallel with the couch. At the limit of this normal though unusual voluntary movement, the joint-play movement is examined at each joint level by moving the vertebra, which is being held, forward, through its interlaminar joints, on the vertebra below it. The posterior part of the movement occurs when the head is carried back to its starting position and allowed to drop back while the vertebra previously being moved is stabilized. The movement now occurs at the interlaminar joints between this and the vertebra above. The examination is started at the occipito-atlantal junction and carried stepwise downward until this movement of joint play is examined for all the interlaminar joints of the cervical spine. Both joints at each level are examined at one time. For the details of technique the reader is referred to Figures 43 and 44. The examiner's left hand is placed behind the neck so as to cradle each dorsal process in the distal inter-

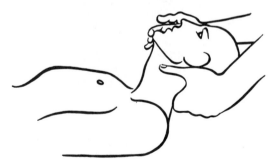

FIGURE 43.   Anteroposterior glide. A position of the head and neck at the end of the anterior aspect of the movement of joint play. The forefinger of the examiner's left hand is thrusting forward and caudalward.

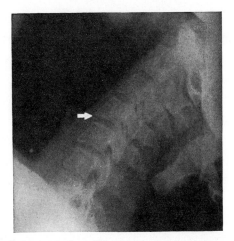

FIGURE 44. Anteroposterior glide. Note position of cervical vertebra at the extreme of the anterior part of the movement. The forward thrust of the examiner's index finger results in a small amount of anterior shift of the fourth cervical vertebra.

phalangeal joint of the index finger. The head is supported in the palm of the left hand and the face is kept horizontal by guiding the chin with the right hand. The index finger is placed behind the spinous process of the first cervical vertebra. The head is lifted anteriorly and at the same time pushed toward the feet.

When the end of this motion can be felt, an additional thrust is applied to the vertebrae through the index finger in a sharp springing motion. The head is then allowed to drop back toward the couch. Just before the head reaches the couch the spinous process of the vertebra is stabilized and the head then allowed to continue backward, thus producing the posterior part of the movement of joint play between the occiput and the atlas. The index finger is then placed to cradle the second spinous process and the head is carried forward again, the examining process being carried on down the spine. Figure 44 demonstrates the effect of the anterior part of this movement between the fourth and fifth cervical vertebrae.

Side Glide. During this examination each vertebra is carried first to one side and then to the other over the vertebra beneath it, thus examining the sidewise movement of joint play of the interlaminar joints between the two vertebrae. The examiner's hands are placed to either side of the head and the occiput cradled in the third, fourth and fifth fingers and the ulnar portion of the palms.

The chin is dropped onto the neck and the head is carried to one side and then the other, keeping the chin and nose parallel with the long axis of the body. Figure 45 shows the way the head

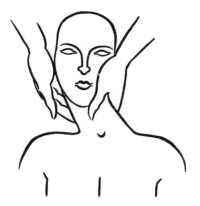

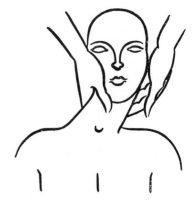

FIGURE 45. The end position of lateral carry to the right. At this point the joint-play movement of side glide is elicited by exerting a thrust to the right by the examiner's left index finger. Note that the vertical position of the head is maintained.

FIGURE 46. The end position of lateral carry to the left. Note the reversal of the part played by the examiner's two hands.

is carried to its limit to the right before the examining manipulative thrust is made. Figure 46 shows the carrying of the head to the left.

If the head is carried to the right, the spinous process of the first cervical vertebra rests on the distal interphalangeal joint of the mobilizing left hand and the transverse process is felt at the proximal interphalangeal joint.

This movement is best controlled when the examiner's forearms are held at a wide angle to the neck. The head is carried to the limit of its range of voluntary movement, when an additional springing thrust is applied through the lateral process of the vertebra which is being held, moving this vertebra slightly to the right on the one below and opening the interlaminar facet joint on the right. Without stopping, the head is then carried to the left by the mobilizing right hand, which applies a thrust through the index finger on the lateral process at the end of the range of voluntary movement. As the head is again carried to the right, the left index finger is moved downward one vertebra, and, at the end of normal movement, the springing thrust is once again utilized to mobilize this vertebra on the one below it and to open the facet joint on the right.

Occipito-atlantal Rock and Rotation. In these movements the large rocker-shaped joints between the occiput and the atlas are examined. A rocking movement here is necessary for the completion of all voluntary movement of the head on the neck. As the patient cannot execute this movement unassisted, it is an involuntary movement at all times. The maneuver to be described is the only safe one to examine this movement.

The head is turned to the right side and the chin is pushed into the shoulder. The occiput is cradled in the fingers and palm of the right hand and lifted from the couch to flatten the cervical spine. The left hand is laid along the line of the left mandible with the palm near the ear and the fingertips on the chin. At the end of voluntary rotation the chin is thrust into the shoulder at the same time that the occiput is slightly lifted and rotated anteriorly. The position of the hands is then exchanged, the occiput being held by the left hand and the right hand being laid upon the right cheek. The head is again lifted and the movement performed toward the left side.

Figure 47A shows the position of the head in full voluntary rotation. Figure 47B shows the position of the examiner's hands superimposed preparatory to producing the joint-play rock at the occipito-atlantal junction which completes the full range of movement of the head on the cervical spine. Figure 48 shows the X-ray appearances of the cervical spine at the limit of voluntary rotation which is the position demonstrated in Figure 47A.

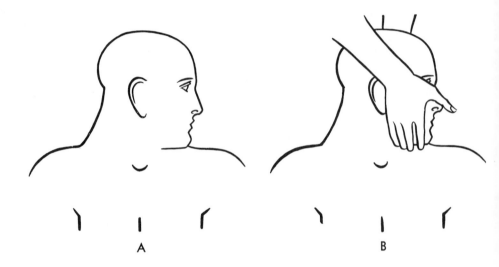

A   B

FIGURE 47. (A) Position of head and neck at the limit of voluntary rotation; (B) with hands superimposed. This is the position adopted at the start of the anterior rocking movement between the occiput and the atlas.

Figure 49A shows the position of the head on the neck on completion of the joint-play rock movement, which can only be safely achieved with a patient in the supine position. Figure 49B shows the examiner's hands superimposed at the limit of the performance of this movement. Figure 50 is an X-ray taken on completion of the rock and should be compared with Figure 48 before the full significance of the movement can be appreciated.

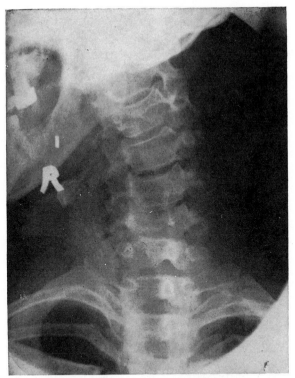

FIGURE 48. Cervical spine at the limit of the movement of voluntary
rotation of the head on the neck.

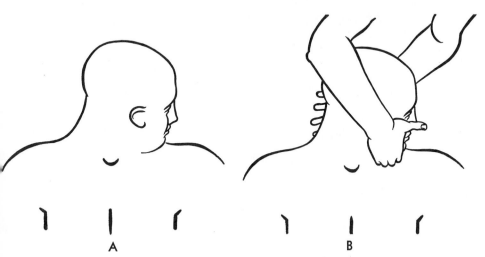

FIGURE 49. (A) Completion of the occipito-atlantal rock; (B) with
examiner's hand superimposed. These drawings show the extent of additional rotation compared with that achieved in Figure 47.

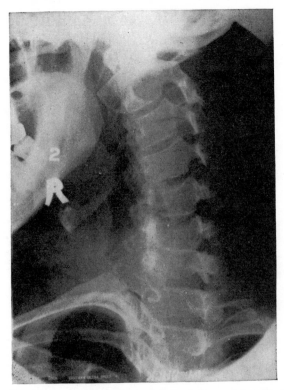

FIGURE 50. Cervical spine on completion of the occipito-atlantal rock.
The relationship of the occiput and mandible should be noted. The
apparent opening of the neural foramina is largely, of course, an optical
illusion.

Side Tilting. This movement side tilts each vertebra on the one
below it to open the interlaminar facet joints individually. To
achieve this the voluntary movement of side bending is employed to take up the slack at each level, at which time the side
tilt can be elicited.

This movement is one of pure side bending of the head and
upper cervical spine. The chin, which lies at a level low on the
cervical spine, scarcely leaves the midline and closely represents
the pivot point of the movement of side tilting.

The degree of side tilt increases at each lower level from the occiput downward to the fourth cervical vertebra, being minimal at the occipito-atlantal junction and maximum at the junction between the third and fourth and fourth and fifth cervical vertebrae, after which its extent again decreases.

The patient's chin is dropped onto the neck. The occiput is cradled in the fingers of the right hand with the palm against the side of the head to move the head to the left in side bending. The spinous and left lateral processes of the first cervical vertebra are cradled in the left forefinger. The left forearm is at a wide angle to the neck, and the right elbow is close beside the examiner's body as the head is tilted to the left. The nose, which represents the surface anatomy of the vertebral pivot about which the movement at this level takes place, overlying the first vertebra, never leaves the midline during this part of the examination. The forehead is moved to the left of the midline and the chin somewhat to the right. When this range of voluntary motion is completed, a short springing thrust is applied by the left index finger against the atlas, while the head is stabilized with the right hand. The occipito-atlas joint on the right is tilted open.

The tilt of the head is then somewhat straightened and the left index finger is carried downward to cradle the processes of the second vertebra and the movement of side-bending of the head is again performed. At the end of this voluntary movement, a thrust is applied to the second vertebra while the head is again stabilized. This time the pivot point on the face is the upper lip, which does not leave the midline. These movements of the head to the left open up the individual joints on the right and actually compress the joints and the discs on the left, which may produce pain should pathology be present in one of these joints or discs.

Figure 51 shows the progressive steps taken to bring the

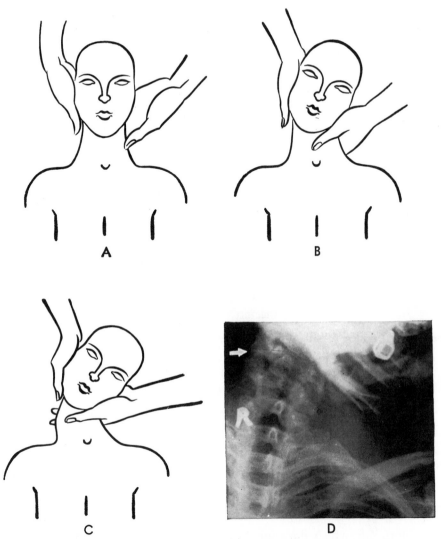

FIGURE 51.   Joint-play movement of side tilting between the fifth and
sixth cervical vertebrae. (A) Starting position. (B) The second step,
consisting of voluntary side bending of the cervical spine. Note that the
position of the examiner's right hand has not changed. (C) Movement
of side tilting completed. Note the position of the head and that the
examiner's right hand has scarcely changed from its position in step two.
The examiner's left hand has thrust toward the midline of the neck.
(D) Cervical spine at completion of the movement of side tilting. Opening up of the joint can be seen.

subject into position to elicit the side tilt at the right interlaminar joint between the fifth and sixth cervical vertebrae. Figure 51A shows the starting position. Figure 51B shows the position when the slack has been taken up, prior to exerting the examining manipulative thrust. Figure 51C shows the position at the end of the manipulative thrust and Figure 51D shows the localized opening of the right interlaminar joint between the fifth and sixth cervical vertebrae.

Palpation

To complete the examination of the neck, palpation of the base of the skull should be done and clinically there may be found localized areas of acute tenderness at the nuchal line to the right and left of the midline.

These tender areas are remarkably constant when there is pathology involving the odontoid process joint and the junctions between the atlas and axis and the axis and the third cervical vertebra.

Palpation at the superior vertebral angle of the scapula reveals a curiously constant localized tender spot when pathology is present both at the junction of the sixth and seventh cervical vertebrae and, strangely, between the fourth, fifth and sixth thoracic vertebrae.

Palpation over the middle of the upper border of the trapezius as it flares out into the arm reveals a constant localized tender spot when pathology is present between the fifth and sixth cervical vertebrae.

Palpation of the neck and examination of the upper thoracic spine and upper chest and mediastinum must be made. Also, the pulses of the arms and the blood pressures of each arm must be tested and compared and the axillae must be examined.

Neurological Examination

A neurological examination of the upper limbs must be undertaken, and examination of the eyes for Horner's syndrome (or the reverse of Horner's syndrome).

The tendon reflexes, though being indicative of fairly specific levels of pathology, may be inhibited by voluntary effort and too great a reliance should not be placed on them. The biceps reflex arc passes through the fifth and sixth cervical cord levels; the supinator reflex passes through the same levels; the pronator reflex passes through the sixth cervical level; and the triceps reflex passes through the seventh cervical and first thoracic levels. No reflex arc appears above the fifth cervical level, which leaves much to be desired if one relies upon neurological signs to determine the level of pathology. Loss of muscle power or muscle wasting may be more reliable signs than reflex or sensory deficits. X-ray examination and analysis of the spinal fluid may be very necessary adjuncts to the clinical examination used in making a differential diagnosis between symptoms arising in the cervical spine and symptoms of neurogenic origin.

8

Therapeutic Manipulation

The maneuvers used in therapeutic manipulation are, with one exception, exactly those used in the diagnostic techniques which have been fully described in the preceding chapters. There are two or three additional maneuvers for certain joints which are described later (pages 116–124).

The therapeutic techniques differ from the diagnostic techniques in only one respect: whereas in the diagnostic examination the examining movement stops when the sign of pain is elicited, in therapy the same manipulative maneuver takes the joint through the pain point to the completion of its normal range of movement. For this reason alone it is essential, therefore, for the would-be manipulator not only to be familiar with the normal average range of movement at all joints, but also to become aware of each individual patient's normal range. Usually this is possible to ascertain, because in traumatic cases, even in the back, the joints on one side will be affected while those of the other side will remain normal.

No one should attempt therapeutic manipulation of any joint until he is perfectly facile in his ability to put a normal joint through its normal range of movement; this means practicing on normal subjects. Nor should anyone attempt therapeutic manipulation of a spinal joint until he is adept in his technique of manipulating the more easily handled joints of the extremities.

In practicing on the normal subject, each manipulative movement should be absolutely pain free; if the normal subject experiences any discomfort on the performance of any movement, then the technique of performance of that movement is wrong.

Perhaps the greatest difficulty in explaining the subject of manipulation in writing is that manipulative therapy is an art. The techniques of an art can only be taught with any certainty by practical demonstration. It is my experience that it takes six months for a well-trained physician in preceptorship training on patients and practicing on the normal subject after hours to master the science of diagnosis and the art of therapy, using manipulative methods. Thus, to learn this subject is a formidable undertaking for an active medical practitioner. But if it is worth doing, it is worth doing well. Anything but the use of correct technique places the patient in jeopardy and the reputation of the method will suffer rather than the reputation of the practitioner of the method.

The use of manipulative therapy in medicine is twofold: first, it is used for the relief of pain arising from joint dysfunction; secondly, it is used to restore the range of movement to a joint whose function is impaired. These aims are not synonymous, for it is possible to relieve pain arising in or from a joint without subjectively altering the voluntary range of movement.

Though occasionally one uses movements in the voluntary range of movement in manipulating certain joints of the extremities, no therapeutic manipulation should be concerned with voluntary movement in joints of the spine. All therapeutic movements of the joints of the spine should fall within the range of the movements of joint play.

It must be stressed that the restoration of normal joint function in spinal joints not infrequently relieves symptoms mistakenly diagnosed as arising from the viscera.

Joint dysfunction does not necessarily give rise to pain locally in the joint; joint dysfunction may give rise to a pain symptom at any place which shares a common nerve supply with the joint. It is partially for this reason that manipulative therapy enjoys a spurious reputation in some quarters. It is well recognized that gall bladder disease may produce, as its presenting symptoms, pain at the level of the eighth thoracic vertebra. Coronary artery disease may present pain at the level of the fourth thoracic vertebra, as well as in the left shoulder and arm, and in the jaw. The reverse situations are (1) when dysfunction of the inter-laminar joints between the fourth and fifth thoracic vertebrae gives rise to pain over the precordium, which can easily be mis-diagnosed as pain in the heart, and (2) when dysfunction of the interlaminar joints between the eighth and ninth thoracic verte-brae gives rise to pain over the gall bladder, which can be mis-diagnosed as pain in the gall bladder. These facts are accepted only with the greatest reluctance, if at all. In the case of referred precordial pain, occasionally mistaken for angina, the similarity of the symptom goes further, for the pain from the joint dys-function also is worse with exercise and is relieved by rest just like anginal pain.

There is also the example of confusion between joint dys-function of the right sacroiliac joint and acute appendicitis. These diagnoses may be confused because of the close relation-ship between McBurney's appendix point and Baer's sacroiliac point. The latter, although not more than 1 inch away from the former, is located where the tender anterior sacroiliac joint ligaments can be palpated through the abdominal wall and has nothing at all to do with the possible location of an inflamed appendix.

Thus we find a perfectly reasonable basis in fact for the some-what bizarre stories of miraculous cures by spinal manipulation of all sorts of visceral diseases. Almost invariably the basis of these stories is that the patient has been told a diagnosis which he believes and remembers. If his symptoms are then unrelieved by orthodox treatment, but are later cured by a manipulator, it is not surprising that the patient claims to have been cured of the visceral disease. It does not seem right to conclude that the patient's symptoms must have been neurotic. Neurosis should never be diagnosed except on positive physical signs, any more than any other diagnosis should ever be made without positive physical signs. However, one must not forget that a "neurotic" may develop true pathology and that a normal person who seeks relief of symptoms arising from pathology and fails to find it may develop an overlying anxiety.

Therapeutic manipulation to break intra-articular joint or capsular adhesions in no way differs in technique from that used to restore loss of movement from simple dysfunction. It is true that occasionally in certain joints in the limbs some movement in the voluntary range may be employed to achieve this, but even in the extremities therapeutic manipulation of the joints should be confined to restoring the movements of joint play.

Rules of Manipulation

As with any form of treatment, there are indications and contraindications for joint manipulation. The specific indication for therapeutic manipulation is the presence of joint dysfunction or a loss of a movement or movements in the range of joint play. Contraindications for therapeutic manipulation are the presence of frank bone or joint disease or the absence of joint dysfunction.

A joint usually may safely be manipulated when there is an obvious history of sudden onset of pain at a time of joint stress or strain and when the patient states that rest improves his symptoms. If rest increases joint stiffness and/or the pain in or from the joint, then some inflammatory or disease process should be suspected, and manipulation is contraindicated until these conditions are either ruled out or eradicated. Here it should be remembered that muscle pathology produces the symptoms of increased stiffness following rest. As it is unusual to find joint pathology without muscle pathology in the back, it may be difficult to assess the nature of the underlying joint pathology. In such a case rest of the muscles by support in a flexion cast for a few days, for instance, followed by another clinical examination, may be necessary before deciding whether manipulative therapy is wise or not.

There are certain rules of manipulation which must be observed in treatment if success is to be achieved. No more than one joint should be manipulated at one time; no more than one movement in one joint should be attempted at one time; and only one articular facet of that joint should be moved on the immobilized opposing facet. No abnormal movement must ever be imparted upon the joint being manipulated. No forceful movement must be imparted on it. The manipulative thrust, push or pull should be imparted only after the available "slack" in the joint has been taken up. No assistant should be used; the use of an assistant immediately forfeits the manipulator's absolute control of the manipulative movement. No manipulative movement must be attempted against muscle resistance. The movements of joint play, being involuntary (i.e., not under the control of voluntary muscles) cannot be achieved either by voluntary muscle action or in the presence of protective muscle resistance.

If the manipulator has to try to overcome muscle resistance to produce a manipulative movement, then this movement at once becomes uncontrolled, and probably damaging to the joint. The manipulator must be absolutely relaxed himself or the patient will never relax. Also, if the manipulator is relaxed, it is more likely that his manipulating hands will follow the normal movement of the joint instead of perhaps erroneously trying to make the joint move as his hands wish it to, which may easily produce a harmful abnormal movement.

Use of Anesthesia

Controversy is always great when the subject of the use of joint manipulation with the patient under anesthesia is brought up. It is perfectly safe to use anesthesia so long as no departure is made from the normal manipulative techniques described. It is dangerous to try forcefully to produce a manipulative movement against muscle resistance. Anesthesia is used only to obtain perfect control over a joint by eliminating muscle resistance which cannot be eliminated by other means. It is used to prevent the use of force and not to facilitate it. In my own practice I use anesthesia for an initial therapeutic manipulation in about 20 per cent of cervical, lumbar or sacroiliac joint manipulations and in not more than 5 per cent of thoracic joint manipulations. The anesthetic which I prefer is unadulterated Pentothal following premedication with morphine, 1/4 grain, and atropine, 1/100 grain (in adults), given three-quarters of an hour before the manipulation. I condemn the added use of muscle relaxants, which should never be given without the patient being intubated, which makes a major procedure out of a minor one.

There is an area of the spine which has caused me trouble in manipulating under anesthesia, namely, between the ninth and eleventh thoracic vertebrae. When I have been manipulating the joints at these levels the patient has on occasion stopped breathing for a few moments — too often to be mere coincidence;

the reflex mechanism cannot be explained by reference to the recognized reflex arcs; but the fact should be remembered. It is a startling experience but the embarrassment of respiration is transient. Fortunately anesthesia is seldom required to allow controlled manipulation in the thoracic spine.

The use of local anesthesia is sometimes sufficient to allow the patient to relax adequately for a manipulative procedure to be achieved. The appropriate interspinous ligaments are infiltrated and paravertebral infiltration is used as well in an attempt to instill the local anesthetic into or around the ligaments of the facet joints. When dealing with the sacroiliac joints, it is often sufficient to infiltrate the posterior joint ligaments around the level of the posterior superior iliac spines. When dealing with the cervical joints, it is sometimes necessary to infiltrate trigger areas in the back musculature of the forequarters to obtain relaxation.

It is no more irrational to use anesthesia to provide relaxation and to avoid pain in joint manipulation than it is to use it for the reduction of fractures and dislocations, or, for that matter, extracting a tooth.

Results of Manipulation

Following a therapeutic manipulation, be it performed with or without anesthesia and be it performed for the relief of pain, for the restoration of function or for the breaking of adhesions, the patient should experience immediate relief from the symptoms for which the manipulation was performed. If there is an exacerbation of symptoms or no relief, then either the manipulative technique was wrong or the diagnosis was wrong and the therapy was not indicated. One should be able to predict the outcome of a therapeutic manipulation just as surely as a physician or surgeon in any other branch of medicine can predict the result of therapy.

Additional Manipulative Techniques

Besides the examining techniques which are also used in therapeutic manipulation there are additional techniques for therapy in treating some joints of the spine. The following techniques are never used in examination.

Backward Tilt of Thoracic Interlaminar Joints

The following therapeutic maneuver to produce the backward-tilt movement of joint play at the thoracic intervertebral junctions between the fourth and twelfth vertebrae is often useful.

Crossed-hands Technique. The patient lies in the prone position with the arms in a relaxed position and a pillow under the chest (Fig. 52). The manipulation is started at the lowest level at which symptoms were found on examination and carried upward. The examiner crosses his left wrist over the right one, placing the ulnar borders of the palms as nearly parallel as possible. The hypothenar eminences are then placed on either side of the spinous process of the vertebra, coming to lie, therefore, over the transverse processes of the vertebra. The borders of the palms are kept as close together as possible. At the end of expiration, the springing manipulative thrust is made at right angles to the curve of the spine in the segment involved. In the midthoracic spine, the thrust is directed almost perpendicularly to the table. In the lower spine, the thrust is directed somewhat toward the head of the patient. In the upper thoracic spine, the thrust is directed somewhat toward the feet.

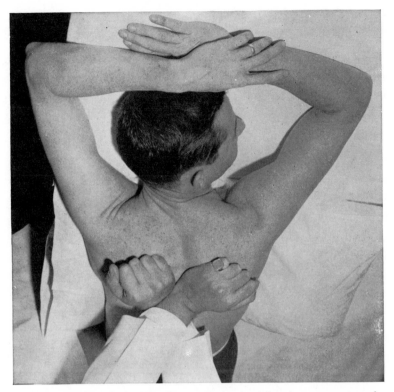

FIGURE 52. Position adopted to perform the joint-play movement of backward tilt at the interlaminar intervertebral joints at the level of the sixth interthoracic junction. The patient lies in the prone position.

Knee-in-the-back Technique. The knee-in-the-back technique is perhaps the most efficient for manipulating joints in the mid-thoracic spine. The joints between the third and ninth thoracic vertebrae can be manipulated using this technique.

In using this technique one of the rules of manipulative therapy is deliberately broken and two movements are performed at one time, namely, long-axis extension and backward tilting. The patient sits on a stool with his back to the physician. The patient's feet should rest comfortably on the floor. Sitting sideways on a chair is adequate though the back of the chair may get in the way. The patient sits far enough forward on the seat to allow the manipulator to put his right foot on the seat. A small pillow is placed between the manipulator's knee and the vertebra which gives rise to the superior facet of the joint which is to be moved. This stabilizes that vertebra and that facet. The patient puts his hands behind his neck, locking his fingers together. The manipulator takes hold of the patient's midforearms by entwining his wrists and hands under the patient's upper arms in the axilla, and then by dorsiflexing his wrists he takes hold of the patient's forearms on their posterior surface. The patient then flops on the manipulator's supporting arms; the elbows hang forward as does the head on the neck. The position is illustrated in Figure 53. The manipulator then lifts the patient through

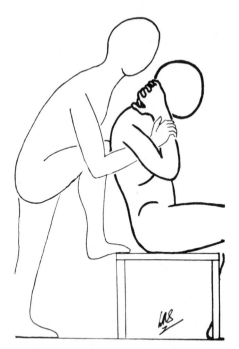

FIGURE 53.   Knee-in-the-back technique. This method produces the movement of joint play, opening up the superior aspect of the inter-laminar intervertebral joints at one level, in this instance the sixth thoracic junction.

his axillae without "winging the arms"; this produces both extension of the thoracic spine and long-axis extension at the joints above the level of the knee in the back. When the slack is taken up, the position is stabilized and by a slight forward thrust of the knee the appropriate vertebra is tilted backward, thereby mobilizing the respective joints at the required level. At no time must the patient's arms be abducted or winged. Figure 54 shows

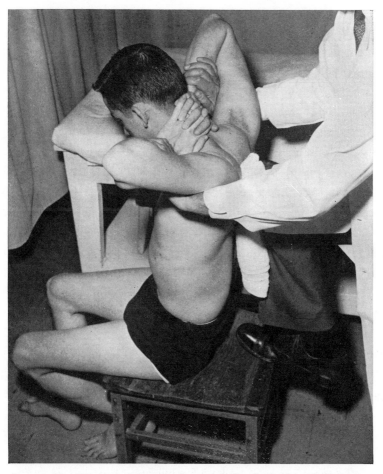

FIGURE 54. Winging of the arms in performing the backward tilt movement between two thoracic vertebrae. This is the wrong way to elicit this movement. Using abnormal forces may hurt the patient severely.

the wrong way of doing this. For the knee to reach the higher vertebrae the patient sits further forward on the stool; for the knee to reach the lower vertebrae the patient's body must be flexed forward from the hips.

In the sitting position, it is sometimes impossible to obtain patient relaxation and an alternative, though slightly less efficient, method of achieving the same thing is performed with the patient standing.

Standing Lift. For the standing maneuvers, the patient stands with his back to the manipulator, who stands with his right side obliquely toward the patient. A small pillow is placed between the manipulator's chest and the vertebra immediately beneath the level of joint dysfunction. The patient puts his right hand on his left shoulder and his left hand on his right shoulder. The manipulator encircles the patient's body with his arms and clasps one of the patient's elbows with his hands. The manipulator then lifts the patient's body weight until he feels that all the slack is taken up and he is about to lift the patient from the floor. The manipulator then lifts a little bit more so that the patient just leaves the floor. This last movement exerts long-axis extension. At the same time he squeezes the patient over the pillow and thrusts forward through the pillow with his chest wall. This produces that backward tilt at the facet joint which is required. For the patient to be relaxed, he must lean his head backward on the manipulator's shoulder and not try to support himself during the lift by coming up on his toes. If his head is unsupported or he comes up on his toes, his erector spinae muscles will immediately contract, making the manipulative movement impossible. Figure 55 shows the position with the lift; Figure 56 shows the unrelaxed position during the lift which will prevent the manipulative maneuver and hurt the patient.

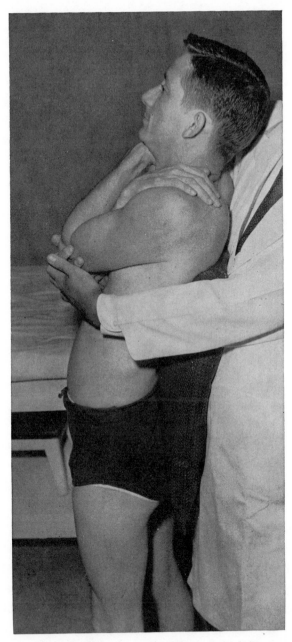

Figure 55. Position adopted to produce the backward tilt movement at a thoracic intervertebral junction when using the standing method. The upper edge of the pillow stabilizes the vertebra just below the joints to be manipulated.

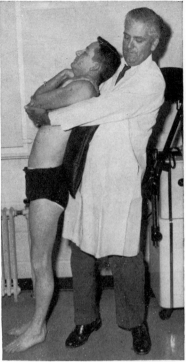

FIGURE 56.   Wrong method in performing the backward tilt movement.
The patient has come up on his toes instead of allowing the examiner to
lift him from the floor; this means that the erector spinae muscles are
in action, preventing the performance of the joint-play movement.

Backward Tilt of Lumbar Interlaminar Joints

Back-to-back Lift. A similar standing maneuver is conveniently used to manipulate the intervertebral joints of the lumbar
spine. The patient and the manipulator stand back to back.
Instead of the pillow, the manipulator's buttocks are used to stabilize the vertebra above the level of the joint which is to be
manipulated. It is surprising how accurately the vertebral level
can be assessed by use of the buttocks. In performing the back-
to-back lift, care must be taken not to hyperextend the lumbar

spine. For the high lumbar levels, or if there is marked disparity in height between manipulator and patient, the manipulator must stand on a stool to adjust his height to that of the patient. The patient rests his head backward on the manipulator. The manipulator then lifts the patient straight up until he feels the patient is about to be lifted up from the floor; this takes up the slack in the joints. He then continues the lift at the same time thrusting backward with the buttocks, obtaining both long-axis extension at the level required and a backward tilt of the vertebra

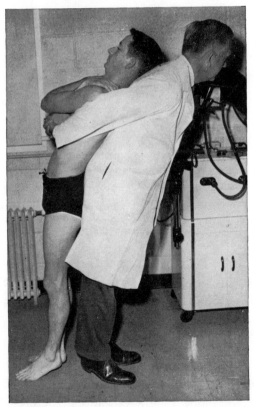

FIGURE 57. Back-to-back lift. This produces the movements of joint play of long-axis extension and backward tilt at the lumbosacral junction.

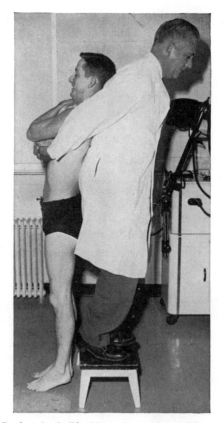

FIGURE 58.   Back-to-back lift. Note change in position adopted by examiner to elicit long-axis extension and backward tilt at higher levels
in the lumbar spine.

through its facet joints. The patient must not come up on his
toes or hold his head forward; if he does, the erector spinae
muscles contract and prevent the movement of joint play which
is being attempted. Each intervertebral level specifically can be
manipulated in this manner from the thoracolumbar through
the lumbosacral levels by proper positioning of the manipulator's
buttocks. Figure 57 shows the position adopted for manipulating
the lumbosacral joints. Figure 58 shows the position adopted for
manipulating the thoracolumbar junction joints.

Aftertreatment

However, let it not be supposed that manipulative treatment is necessarily all that is required to relieve pain arising from the back. It may just be the beginning of a plan of treatment-management. (Also see page 193.)

Maintenance of Normal Movement. Unless the muscles which control the voluntary movements of the spine are ready to resume their normal voluntary control of the joints to which normal function has been restored, dysfunction will readily recur. So, following successful manipulative therapy, it is necessary to maintain the range of movement which has been attained until normal muscle control is reinstituted.

Muscle Re-education and Support. After prolonged secondary muscle spasm with splinting of the joints in which there is pain, the muscles may be so atrophied and weak as to require temporary support while they are being re-educated. A corset, a simple back brace or an abdominal binder may be required. Usually the muscles which are weakened by atrophy from prolonged spasm in the back are those of the erector spinae group and symmetrical back extension exercises should be prescribed. It is usually obvious on clinical examination that it is the extensor muscles of the back that are affected by back pathology and it is these muscles which require strengthening after the causative pathology of back pain has been removed. Re-education of the abdominal muscles may be important as they are the anterior supporting muscles of the spine. Though exercises to achieve this may flex the spine they should not be thought of as spine flexion exercises.

If any form of back support is used in the convalescent period, the patient must be warned that continued use of the support will further weaken the muscles and that it is being prescribed as a temporary measure only. No pressure pads should ever be incorporated into such a support as pressure over muscle will produce atrophy in it. To support the low back adequately, the apparatus must have a belt which can be worn horizontally and tightly around the pelvis, with its upper edge hooked under the anterior superior spine. This belt should not be more than 2 inches in width and it should not be shaped in any manner.

Skin Rolling and Effleurage. If there has been marked tightness and tenderness on skin rolling as a result of spinal pathology, restoration of joint function can do nothing to overcome this and the tight tender skin and fascia may become a primary cause of secondary joint dysfunction. This can be avoided only by treatment directed at loosening the "panniculo-fibrositis." This is achieved by the therapy of skin rolling and is best done following the application of superficial heat — infrared radiation seems to be the most satisfactory method of application. The skin rolling, which is painful and tends to set up reflex muscle spasm, must be followed by effleurage for as long as it takes to achieve muscle relaxation. The effleurage will also disperse the congestion of the tissues resulting from the heat which, left alone, may set up reflex muscle spasm.

Rest. Following the relief of joint dysfunction, especially of long standing, the use of rest cannot be too highly stressed. And in this context rest means rest from function or weight bearing, not from movement. Movement must be maintained. I have never found it necessary to use a bed board for patients with joint dysfunction so long as the bed mattress is firm (not hard). In fact most patients with back pain are more comfortable in the semi-Fowler's position than flat on a bed board.

Posture. Following manipulation of the joints of the low back and especially the sacroiliac joints, the patient must never be allowed to sit with the legs stretched out straight in front of him. Such a position is in fact the position used in performing the straight-leg-raising tests. From the description of these tests it will be remembered that straight-leg-raising exerts a backward torsion strain on the sacroiliac joints and, when both are raised together, not only on these joints but on those at the lumbosacral junction as well. So, to let a patient sit with his legs outstretched in the convalescent period is as much to be avoided as any deliberate attempt to cause a recurrence of trouble.

Adjunctive Treatment. A more detailed correlation of treatment-management for back pain will be found in Chapter 13, which deals with the correlation of pathology and treatment in whiplash injuries. Almost all traumatic pathology in the back arises from a type of whiplash injury, as, for that matter, do traumatic joint conditions in the extremities. The basis of joint dysfunction is usually that the patient's joint(s) is subjected to an unguarded movement during the performance of a normal voluntary movement. In Chapters 10 through 12 adjunctive treatment to manipulative therapy for traumatic low back pain is considered, the treatment, of course, being dictated by the differential diagnosis. This is included because the patient's symptoms often do not arise solely from joint dysfunction, and treatment of the patient must fail if only one of the etiological factors is corrected. It is often because the secondary etiological factors are ignored by osteopaths in their treatment that their otherwise excellent manipulative procedures fail where they might be expected to succeed.

9

Prophylactic Treatment Against Joint Dysfunction in the Spine

It is very likely that bad habits in posture and in the use of the back which are acquired during the growth years predispose to faulty use of the spinal joints and subsequent dysfunction in later life. Fortunately the average person develops normally, and normal resilience in the joints of the spine is sufficient to allow for the back's adaptation to normal activity without symptoms from dysfunction arising. But there are many people who suffer from the back pain of dysfunction who might have been spared much suffering if some attention had been paid to their backs early in life.

Posture

Postural training at home and in physical education classes at school should be the beginning of prophylactic treatment against joint dysfunction in the back. However, the usual demands of parents and teachers too often tend to teach bad, rather than good, habits of stance and the use of the back.

The common admonition to a child to stand up straight, to pull his shoulders back, to keep his chin up, to throw his chest out and to pull his tummy in could not be better calculated to produce abnormal postural stresses on his spinal joints.

129

Good posture too often is considered to be a static phenomenon, whereas in fact it should be a dynamic one. Any method of postural training which stresses static posturing defeats its own purpose. Static occupational postures most surely give rise to pain from dysfunction in the spinal joints; common examples of this are the typist, who suffers from pain in the upper third of the thoracic spine, and the surgeon, who after a long surgical procedure suffers pain from dysfunction in both the upper thoracic and the low lumbar spine.

Normal good posture in the standing position is achieved in a relaxed person who holds his head up with the chin drawn in, the arms stretching down toward the floor and the buttocks slightly contracted. Normal good posture in the sitting position is achieved by placing the buttocks so that they just touch the back of the seat being used. Then, on sitting upright, the spine adopts its normal posture without further drill. Normal good posture in bed is achieved by the use of a firm, not hard, mattress which maintains the normal spine contours at rest.

Disease and Posture. The slouch of a child suffering from adenoids and asthma cannot be corrected by fatiguing postural back exercises. In the adenoidal child, if the airway is cleared by the removal of the hypertrophied tissue, and if he is taught to breathe properly, his posture will improve spontaneously. The improvement may well be enhanced because a potent debilitating focus of infection has been removed and the child's ready fatiguability from chronic absorption of toxins no longer produces postural faults caused by tiredness. In the asthmatic child, postural faults will rapidly improve when he is taught to breathe properly.

Persistent abnormal posture in a child may be due to structural congenital anomalies or to congenital or developmental diseases. It is remarkable, however, how seldom these patients complain of pain, so much so that any child who does complain of back pain should receive the most serious attention and a most thorough diagnostic work-up, as back pain in a child usually heralds serious disease.

Poor posture may result from fatigue due to malnutrition or to incipient systemic disease; these factors must be checked before blaming faulty mechanics or attributing the defect to laziness.

That postural faults in children and adolescents may indicate psychological maladjustment is undoubtedly true. In such patients, it should be clear that postural exercises can do nothing to correct the primary problem and insistence on them may aggravate the situation. Nor should blindness or deafness be forgotten as causes of postural deviations which will not respond to physical treatment alone.

Footwear and Posture. The heel height of footwear has a great bearing on the postural curves of the spine. This subject has been discussed at some length (pages 51–52 and pages 64–65). Normally, the spinal joints will not be painful at rest, i.e., standing with normal relaxed posture, if their articular facets are in their normal anatomical relationship to one another. Alteration of the normal spinal curves, which alters the articular facet relationship, occurs with tendo Achillis insufficiency or by wearing too high shoe heels, or by structural alteration of the vertebrae from any cause. Then dysfunction and pain ensue. Poor posture in itself does not give rise to symptoms of pain in the back. It is only when dysfunction in the synovial joints supervenes that symptoms occur.

Individual variations from "normal" may be normal for an individual and, as such, must not be confused with the abnormal. For this reason, classes for postural remedial exercises should be regarded with suspicion unless each member of the class receives individual attention from the instructor as needed.

Physical educators would be better advised to teach their students efficient use of what bodies they have, rather than to make often useless and sometimes harmful attempts at developing what is regarded as the ideal body. If children were taught to lift properly, using their legs instead of their backs, to avoid twisting and stooping, and to maintain their anterior spinal supports, i.e., their abdominal muscles, in good order, it is probable that the incidence of back problems in later life would be very much less.

Household Hints. Domestic science teachers would do their students a great service if they would include in their courses of instruction methods of sparing the back in everyday living. The use of a high stool at the sink or at the ironing board provides incalculable benefit to all housewives, as does use of a ladder when reaching down heavy objects from high cupboards or hanging up clothes. Bed-making, turning mattresses, moving furniture, carrying groceries, lifting babies and such everyday chores can all be done in a right or wrong way; and the wrong way often leads to the onset of back pain from joint dysfunction.

When there is no underlying structural anomaly, systemic disease, malnutrition or other cause of easy fatiguability, or psychological hindrance, poor posture can be treated by various exercise programs, which so long as they are dynamic and not static will maintain joint mobility and prevent dysfunction and pain from so-called postural joint strain.

Prophylaxis Following Dysfunction

Later in life, when dysfunction has occurred and has been relieved by manipulation, prescribed exercises should maintain normal function in the affected joints. However, patients tend to do exercises only so long as they remember their pain. Yet once they stop their exercises, dysfunction is likely to recur. This can largely be prevented by prophylactic manipulation to maintain normal mobility in the joints. I instruct my patients to return for such treatment if they feel themselves tightening up. This "tightening up" is often the prodromal symptom of dysfunction.

Prophylaxis Post-partum

Many women develop low back pain in the post-partum period. Commonly, their symptoms arise because one or both of their sacroiliac joints are lax at this time. The injury to these joints, which is the cause of their pain, is usually that of backward subluxation. It is caused either (1) when the patient is delivered in the dorsal position, with the legs held in stirrups in unnatural flexion, especially if the labor is long and the bearing down vigorous; or (2) when the patient is allowed to sit up in bed after delivery with the legs outstretched, i.e., without the knees being flexed. The mechanism of the joint injury is that the hamstring muscles pull unduly from their ischial origins, rotating the os innominatum of one or both sides backward on the sacrum through the sacroiliac joint(s). This may be unnoticed so long as the joints are lax, but if they involute in this position, a fixed backward subluxation results.

Prophylactic treatment against back pain from these causes requires delivery in one or another of the side-lying positions in routine cases. This obviously lessens the chances of sacroiliac subluxation, and does not increase the difficulty of delivery. In the lying-in period, the mother should never sit up in bed without the knees being flexed by suitable adjustment of the bed. The use of a many-tailed binder, properly applied, will help to prevent abnormal joint movement. The lowest part of the binder should be around the hips and horizontally around the body just below the anterior superior iliac spines. There are systems of post-partum exercises which, when adequately taught and performed, restore abdominal and perineal muscle tone much more efficiently than when the process is left to chance; these exercises are prophylactic against post-partum back pain.

Prophylaxis Following Surgery

Flat back strain, which occurs in the postoperative patient who has been subjected to prolonged surgery under deep anesthesia, could be avoided were more attention paid to the positioning of patients on the operating table. It occurs because no operating table has yet been designed to support the lumbar lordosis. In the third stage of anesthesia, the muscles cease their supportive function, and gravity exerts forces to flatten the lumbar spine to the flat surface of the operating table. As the patient recovers from the anesthetic and the erector spinae muscles regain their tone, the lumbar vertebrae may be locked in this flattened position, unless by movement or other good fortune the vertebrae regain their normal lordotic arrangement. Prophylactic treatment against flat back strain is either to keep the patient's knees slightly flexed while he is on the operating table, or to place a very small pillow under the lumbar spine to support its lordosis before the patient is anesthetized. A small pneumatic pillow, built into the operating table, and inflated before the patient is anesthetized so that he can tell when the support is adequate, would be an ideal prophylactic measure.

The vigorous "manipulative" maneuvers to which the cervical spine is subjected by some anesthetists while they intubate a patient are potent causes of postoperative neck pain. Controlled manipulation of the cervical spinal joints is considered by many to be dangerous, especially under anesthesia, yet the contortions through which the neck is put by some anesthetists fail to alarm them.

The careless positioning of an anesthetized patient on the operating table and the callous way in which assistants sometimes transfer these patients from the operating table to a stretcher or back to bed are also potential causes of postoperative back pain from traumatic joint strain and dysfunction. The prophylactic measures to prevent this are more careful supervision of anesthetic procedures and of operating room assistants in their care of patients.

Postoperatively, no patient should ever be allowed to get up without first putting on his normal walking shoes. To shuffle around in heelless bedroom slippers, especially after abdominal or back surgery, frequently promotes back pain. This subject is discussed again in Chapter 11 (page 192).

The importance of retraining the abdominal wall muscles in their supportive functions after abdominal surgery cannot be too highly stressed as a prophylactic measure against postoperative back pain, just as it is important to retrain the erector spinae muscles after back surgery or therapeutic manipulation. This subject is considered at some length in Chapter 11 (page 193). Postoperative, post-partum and postmanipulative patients must also be taught good habits in the use of their backs, and must avoid stooping, twisting and heavy lifting until their musculature has regained its normal supportive and functional standards.

Though most surgeons know that the use of supportive pillows under a lower limb stump, following amputation, is absolutely contraindicated, nurses still place them under the stumps for *their* patient's comfort. Flexion contractures at the hip rapidly ensue, and if uncorrected are another potential cause of back pain. For the same reason — comfort — pillows are placed under the elbow of patients following chest surgery on the side of the surgical procedure. This has been one of the commonest causes of postsurgical deformity and pain in the back especially following thoracoplasty but also after any chest surgery to a greater or lesser degree. Postoperative physical therapy following chest surgery is the best prophylaxis against cervical and thoracic spine pain. This should consist of suitable breathing exercises and upper limb exercises. After radical mastectomy the same principles should be followed to avoid upper back pain.

Prophylaxis in the Bedridden Patient

Good posture in bed for any patient whether medical or surgical is prophylactic against back pain from joint dysfunction. A patient lying in bed should be moved, or encouraged to move, turning frequently from side to side, lying on the back and, when possible, on the stomach. The sheets should never be tightly tucked in at the foot of the bed; if they are, the feet are held in exaggerated plantar flexion and insufficiency of the Achilles tendons rapidly occurs. This is an irreversible change, and later becomes a potential cause of back pain. To avoid the discomfort of tight sheets, the patient often lies with his legs in external rotation. In this position the iliotibial bands rapidly lose their elasticity, becoming pathologically taut and a potential cause of back pain.

Straining on a bed pan subjects the spinal joints to grossly abnormal stresses, and care of a patient's bowel habits thus becomes a prophylactic measure against back pain from joint dysfunction.

When a patient has improved to the extent that he is allowed to sit up in bed, the knees must be flexed and a small pillow should be placed so as to support the lumbar spine. Too often a pillow (and a large one at that) is placed behind the patient's head, thrusting it forward on the neck. This not only tends to give rise to pain from joint dysfunction in the cervical spine, but also tends to make the patient slump down in bed, with his spine adopting an atavistic curve. If this is uncorrected, back pain will surely result. The cervical lordosis should be supported by a very small pillow, but this should not be placed behind the head.

Nursing and Prophylaxis

In these days when the wonder drugs have almost done away with the art of nursing, the nurse tends to become a pill-pusher and an executive secretary. This is a deplorable situation for, with the loss of the art of nursing, day to day nursing care has become neglected.. One of the most important prophylactic measures against back pain, therefore, is the reinstitution of undergraduate and postgraduate instruction in proper patient care, which means so much to the bedridden patient at all times; but it also may mean much to the future comfort of the individual long after he has given up his patient status.

Of course, nurses alone are not to blame for all these things. Present-day medical training must share the blame too. In too many medical schools, the resident staff is just as ignorant of these first principles of patient care. As the young doctor scales the ladder of his postgraduate training program, he becomes more and more of a prima donna, doing only the heroic part of necessary treatment and leaving the "scut work" care of the patient to the more junior man, who in turn will often leave it to the student. Less and less the attending staff attend to anything except the didactic teaching, and again the art of patient care tends to be overlooked. Of course, in the old days the student picked up much of this art from his everyday contact with efficient nurses. But in the long run, teaching efficient patient care is the responsibility of the man at the top of the medical echelon, and today he is often the only one who has ever seen or known the real importance of good nursing care.

Muscle Training and Prophylaxis

To undertake unaccustomed exercise without training is courting symptoms from muscles and joints in the back. If, in addition, such activity is indulged in when an intercurrent infection is present, serious trouble may ensue. The frequency with which ankylosing spondylitis starts in an athletic type of young man, who is allowed to compete in some sports event, even though it is obvious that he is suffering from an upper respiratory tract infection, cannot be explained by coincidence. To see acute hematogenous osteomyelitis start in a similar way once is to see it once too often. And "unaccustomed activity" should be read to mean not only athletic activity, but also do-it-yourself tasks which require undue effort. Overfatigue, especially in the presence of intercurrent infection, may lead to chronic bone and joint disease, which may be more serious when exposure to dampness is added to the joint and muscle insult.

Lack of training before undertaking some special activity causes unsynchronized movement, which precipitates joint dysfunction. In addition, there also may be a component of traumatic arthritis and synovitis among the etiological factors of the resulting symptom complex. Overfatigue will add to the severity of the resulting pathological conditions.

So, training and the avoidance of unaccustomed exercise become important factors of prophylaxis against back pain.

Prophylaxis and Heat and Cold

The control and placement of air conditioning vents has recently presented problems pertaining to the back. Acute back pain from cold fibrositis and the resulting dysfunction has occurred from improper positioning of this comfort of modern times. Attention to the location of air conditioners and their chilling effect has a place in prophylaxis against back pain. Conversely, overwork in excessive heat, resulting in salt depletion by undue sweating, may present just as great a problem, with muscle cramps and joint dysfunction resulting. Thus salt and water balance also plays a part in prophylaxis against back pain.

Some of the foregoing comments on prophylaxis may seem over-sedulous, but any measure which can lessen the incidence of backache merits the closest scrutiny and should be practiced whenever possible.

10

Conditions Coexisting with Dysfunction Complicating Diagnosis, and Their Treatment

Trauma to the back, regardless of severity, seldom causes simple, localized pathology, and symptoms from back injuries are therefore seldom simple or limited to one anatomical locale. Consideration of the causes of back pain which complicate cases of joint dysfunction and may produce residual symptoms after it has been corrected is important. These same pathological conditions may occur alone without bone, joint or disc pathology and must be recognized as possible primary causes of pain. Having diagnosed these associated conditions as etiological factors in the symptomatology, their treatment must be effective.

At first glance, some of these conditions may appear to be hypothetical. Yet these diagnoses are, for the most part, accepted as causes of symptoms in the extremities, so it should be logical to accept them as causes of symptoms in the back where identical anatomical structures are surely subject to the same pathological changes. Then it is not surprising that the physical signs resulting from these pathological states in the back are, if properly ana-

140

lyzed, identical with those from the same causes in the limbs. Even then the diagnoses must sometimes be arrived at more by logical inference from the signs than by actual demonstration of something visible and palpable.

Traumatic Synovitis

Symptoms of acute traumatic synovitis of a joint come late, after a period of relatively little pain following the traumatic episode. This silent period may be as long as 24 hours. The patient with synovitis of a limb joint may wake the next day to find the involved joint warm, painful, stiff, and swollen. The symptoms are aggravated by any attempt to use (not necessarily to move) the joint. Rest relieves the pain, but the joint becomes stiff. On examination the symptoms can be confirmed as signs, and in addition, some muscle atrophy occurs. The symptoms are identical in traumatic synovitis of a joint of the back. The warmth and swelling of the joint usually cannot be detected by ordinary means, but may be inferred logically; the temperature change could be detected by the use of thermocouples. There may be signs of radiculitis from irritation of the nerve root by pressure from the swelling. Pain and stiffness in the joint can be demonstrated and protective muscle spasm can be seen, which if prolonged, leads to muscle atrophy, particularly of the muscles in the erector spinae groups.

Treatment. Treatment of acute traumatic synovitis is the same whether it be in the joint of a limb or the back. Rest from use of the joint is the crux of successful treatment. Rest from use, however, does not mean rest from movement. Movement without use is the second most important phase of treatment, but movement of the joint must be passive and movement of its supporting and activating muscles must not bring the joint into use. Such muscle movements are called muscle-setting exercises. If the joint is allowed to remain immobile, dysfunction almost certainly results. If the muscles are allowed to remain inactive, atrophy will certainly occur which will later have to be corrected, thus prolonging convalescence unnecessarily.

The use of a bed board and leg traction which keeps the patient lying flat and immobile invalidates these principles of treatment and may increase the symptoms. A firm — not rigid — mattress should be used. Anyone who doubts that a bed board may be harmful should lie flat on a wooden floor without any support of the lordosis of the lumbar and cervical spines and without moving for 20 minutes. The acute back pain which results, especially in the lumbar spine, should be convincing that the prescription of a bed board should not be routine. Similarly, anyone who has undergone prolonged leg surgery under local anesthesia will support this contention. The most comfortable bed position for the patient is the semi-Fowler's position with small pillows supporting the lordosis of the lumbar and cervical spines and with the knees flexed.

When the patient has been made as comfortable as possible by positioning in bed, suitable physical therapy must be prescribed. Heat by the use of hydrocollator pads or hot packs is comforting and relaxing. Infiltration of a local anesthetic around the affected joint gives some temporary comfort.

The joints in the affected area of the back should be moved by the therapist within their *painless* range of voluntary movement.

The muscles must be moved without producing joint function. Muscle-setting exercises are difficult to teach to a patient with pain in the back, but with patience and care it can be done. The faradic current, always hand surged, is also helpful.

The program of physical therapy finishes with the prescription of effleurage (stroking massage). This form of massage helps to disperse edema in the part being treated. It also restores muscle relaxation, which has very likely been lost to some extent during the joint and muscle phases of treatment.

Each phase of treatment is graduated in intensity to the patient's tolerance, which should increase almost daily. As passive movement becomes tolerated in the full range of joint movement and muscle exercise, it is gradually replaced by active movement without function, and finally function may be resumed. Before this can occur any joint dysfunction which may have supervened must be corrected by manipulation.

With regard to the resumption of activity, there can be no doubt that it can be greatly hastened by exercise under water in a Hubbard tank or pool.

The use of ultrasound is probably contraindicated in the treatment of synovitis. There are many who believe that the removal of synovial fluid from a joint hastens recovery from traumatic synovitis. I cannot subscribe to this theory and in fact believe that the aspiration of the fluid may be harmful. It certainly is not necessary as it is when blood or pus is present, and there is always a chance of introducing infection into the joint. The outpouring of synovial fluid into a joint following trauma must be Nature's way of protecting the delicate articular cartilage. Synovial fluid, being normal to a joint, is reabsorbed from it normally once the need for its protective excess quantity is over. It remains so long as its protective qualities are required. Accordingly, if excess synovial fluid does not disappear with treatment, either the diagnosis of the pathology is wrong or the treatment is wrong or both. Aspiration of synovial fluid, then, removes the best clinical sign that we have of the accuracy of our diagnosis and the efficacy of our treatment. So long as excess synovial fluid remains in a joint, so long must functional activity of the joint be restricted. I believe that if this tenet were adhered to in cases of traumatic joint pathology there would be a remarkable drop in the incidence of osteoarthritis in later years.

Hemarthrosis

Symptoms of hemarthrosis are that following the immediate pain of the injury there are worsening of the pain which is not relieved by rest, immediate heat and swelling of the joint, and loss of the ability to use the joint. In hemarthrosis of a joint in the back the history is the same as for traumatic synovitis, but the traumatic episode is more severe. The swelling of hemarthrosis is never so profound as that of synovitis, so it is unlikely that any nerve root signs will develop. The heat of the joint is greater than with synovitis and may be detectable. The protective muscle spasm is more severe than with synovitis and cannot be relieved by positional relaxation. The associated loss of joint movement is also more absolute and involves the joints of neighboring spinal segments, in which there may well be synovitis.

Treatment. Treatment of acute hemarthrosis is similar to that detailed for synovitis, but because the pain of this condition is far greater, the bed-rest position may be impossible to achieve. In such cases nothing short of a plaster bed will bring comfort to the patient.

It is well known that the pain of hemarthrosis is readily relieved by aspiration of the blood from the joint. In fact, this is a most necessary part of treatment to avoid damage to the articular cartilage and the formation of intra-articular adhesions following the absorption of the hematoma. Aspiration of a facet joint is virtually impossible technically. It is in such cases, therefore, that I believe treatment by ultrasound may be helpful.

The likelihood of intra-articular adhesions forming during the period of absorption and healing is greater than with synovitis, and painful dysfunction will occur. Therefore the need for manipulative therapy in this condition before all the symptoms resolve is much more probable.

It is probable that ultrasound increases the permeability of a semipermeable membrane, and the dispersal of an accumulation of fluid within a joint capsule is hastened by its use. It is more effective if given after the application of heat.

In the treatment of any acute back pain it is foolhardy to deny the benefit of sedative or narcotic drugs and they should be used as required. But, I find little use for the muscle relaxant drugs. Their use is usually directed at a secondary condition and adequate physical therapy can be more efficacious.

Contusions of the Soft Tissues

The history of the traumatic episode is clear. The symptoms from painful soft tissue contusions of the back may be severe. The back tends to stiffen with rest. Joint movement is not limited, though there may be severe muscle spasm after moving around.

Treatment. The symptoms respond readily to heat, local anesthetic infiltration and effleurage. Adequate rest for the injured part can usually be obtained by simple support.

For supporting the low back in cases in which traumatic pathology is limited to the soft tissues, I use a method of strapping for which I make no claim of originality, though I am unable to give proper credit to its originator, whoever he may be.

Overlapping lengths of 2-inch adhesive tape are used. They must be long enough to encircle the back from in front of the midaxillary line on each side. The lowest tape should adhere anteriorly just below the anterior superior iliac spines and is the first one to be applied.

The tapes are covered, except at their ends, with 2-inch gauze bandage to keep them from adhering to the skin except at their ends. It is the circumferential tightness and not the area of adherence which provides the efficient support.

A second pelvic band tape is then cut, and to it are stuck the bases of about twelve cotton-tipped applicator sticks. This is then applied over the lowest part of the original strapping. Further unprotected, overlapping 2-inch strips of adhesive tape are applied over the sticks and covering the first layer of tapes.

The whole application is made with the patient lying prone and relaxed. Each tape is started from alternate sides, and the buttocks and flanks of the trunk are pulled up toward the spine from the side away from that on which each tape is initially anchored. This excellent support will last 3 or 4 days, which is usually long enough for its purpose, and heat can be applied through it.

Acute Muscle Tears

A muscle tear may complicate a contusive injury. The symptoms of the tearing of muscle fibers may be those of acute pain localized poorly, but obviously, to an area where anatomically there is chiefly soft tissue. There are two especially common sites in the low back in which muscle tears occur with relatively minor trauma. These are (1) where the erector spinae group of muscles join to their common tendon just above and medial to the posterior superior iliac spines, and (2) at the gluteal origin on the ala of the ilium just lateral to the posterior superior iliac spines. In the history the patient often says that "it felt as though something tore in my back," at the time of the injury. On examination, it is usual to feel a localized, exquisitely tender gathering of fibers in the muscle on palpation. The diagnosis is certain if on bringing the muscle into active contraction, either voluntarily or by faradic stimulation, the pain becomes more intense. Severe local spasm occurs in a muscle in which there are torn fibers.

Treatment. Treatment of torn muscle fibers involves rest from function, but movement without function is important. The support described above (page 146) often suffices to rest the muscle, but bed rest may be needed, and then physical therapy should be directed at maintaining muscle movement. Infiltration of the damaged muscle area with a local anesthetic breaks the pain cycle and allows the damaged muscle to relax. The healing process depends on adequate circulation, and it should be remembered that the blood flow through a muscle depends for its efficiency upon the physiological pumping action of the muscle. This is always lost when a muscle is in spasm, from whatever cause. Another reason for keeping a muscle moving while healing is taking place is that during the healing process formation of scar tissue occurs. Scar tissue contracts, and after this has occurred every movement of the muscle, on resumption of activity, pulls on the scar. This not only interferes with the smooth action of the muscle, but may produce pain from further inflammatory reaction around it. Scar tissue may become adherent to the adjacent uninjured muscle layers with a similar result. One also postulates nerve fibrils being caught up in the contracted scar tissue as a cause of pain. The maintenance of movement in the muscle tends to minimize both the contraction and adherence potentialities.

Chronic Muscle Tears

The symptoms from a healed muscle tear resulting in interference with the normal action of the muscle (pulling on the
scar and adherence of the scar) are a dull aching pain in the
muscle aggravated by exercise, and stiffening in the back with
rest. On examination the muscle tenderness is not well localized
and, in addition, there may be sensitive fibrositic deposits
throughout the muscle involved. In the next section an attempt
is made to account for muscle pain which is commonly attributed to fibrositis. If there is an infective element to the fibrositic
reaction, then treatment first must be directed at eradicating the
focus of infection.

Treatment. Local treatment of the painful scar area aims at
freeing the scar from any adherence and at breaking up the scar
itself. This is achieved by the age-old method of needling, made
more tolerable today by the injection of a local anesthetic. The
area is traumatized by needling, and is then treated as though
there had been a recent muscle tear. Following the initial needling, the patient may experience an exacerbation of symptoms
after the local anesthetic wears off. He should always be warned
of this, and the application of heat locally together with administration of 10 grains of aspirin, maybe with ½ grain of
codeine, is sufficient to alleviate this.

The use of ultrasound, by softening the scar tissue, may be
sufficient to relieve symptoms.

Fibrositis

The diagnosis of fibrositis, which is synonymous with the
terms fibromyositis and myositis, may mean anything or nothing.

It should be used to describe the condition of diffuse infiltration of the soft tissues with areas which are painful on palpation; in some areas, indeed, painful nodules may be felt; hence, the expression "painful deposits." No one, I believe, has ever demonstrated in these nodules a specific pathological entity; the only histological change demonstrated has been nonspecific local areas of round cell infiltration. For this reason, many authorities refuse to recognize the condition as a pathological entity and ascribe the symptoms to psychosomatic upset.

Clinically, however, there can be no doubt that such a condition exists. The symptoms and signs with which it is associated are remarkably constant. The symptoms and signs can be relieved equally constantly by suitable physical therapy without any overt psychotherapy being added to the treatment program.

It is conceivable that, in our way of life, many times a day we lay undue stress or strain on our muscles here and there sufficient to cause minute muscle fiber tears. These are most likely to occur in the muscles of the back and especially in the extensor groups, which are the least trained and probably the most abused muscles in the body. Such tears have to involve macroscopic areas of muscle before they can give rise to symptoms; nonetheless, where fibers are torn, their healing takes place sometimes by regeneration, but more often by laying down fibrous scar tissue. Usually the scarring is probably insufficient to cause inefficiency in muscle action and no symptoms ensue. Now, if joint dysfunction or any other cause of muscle spasm is superimposed, muscle relaxation becomes impaired.

Anything which interferes with physiological relaxation of muscle will start a vicious cycle of events; lack of relaxation produces fatigue, which produces muscle spasm, producing further impairment of relaxation, more fatigue, more spasm, and so on. The flow of venous blood and lymph away from a muscle depends on perfect relaxation and contraction of the muscle. Without relaxation, there are accumulations of lymph and an abnormal degree of venous stasis in the muscle. With accumulation of tissue fluid, there follows an accumulation of catabolites. The waste products of metabolism (lactic acid, notably) are noxious, and where there is any accumulation, an inflammatory reaction develops. Pain ensues in scattered places, especially where pre-existing traumatized areas are present. Pain being added to the vicious cycle produces more spasm and more stasis in the affected muscles.

This is my concept of fibrositis, and this mechanism goes on throughout our active hours. The process can only be reversed by achieving relaxation and restoring normal drainage of the muscles affected. Thus, rational prescription of physical treatment can be expected to relieve the symptoms of the pathology.

Even when the cause of the impaired relaxation is psychological tension, the resulting muscle spasm produces local changes with physical manifestations which cannot be treated by psychological methods alone.

Infective Fibrositis. If to all this is added transient bacteremia or toxemia from any focus of infection in the body, such as an abscess, an infected tooth, pelvic inflammatory disease, etc., infection may smoulder in the ripe medium of the damaged tissue. Thus occurs infective fibrositis. Treatment in this instance will be ineffectual unless the focus of infection is first eradicated.

Cold Fibrositis. Local chilling may produce an acute attack of fibrositis ("cold in the muscle"). In this instance, besides the cycle of changes described above, there is some local spastic effect on the blood vessels, causing local ischemia which may

give rise to severe pain. Treatment, of course, must include removal of the cause, which in this instance is easily counteracted
by the application of heat alone.

Electrolyte Imbalance. A further cause of back pain, which
occurs in hot weather in laborers and manual workers, merits
consideration. Stoker's cramps and miner's cramps are well-
recognized pathological entities due to sodium chloride loss by
excessive sweating. The resulting electrolytic imbalance produces
changes in muscle metabolism resulting in these cramps. In our
unhealthy way of living, it is surprising how deficient the average
person is in his daily fluid intake. Then with excessive exercise
in unusual heat, and with excessive fluid and salt loss due to perspiration, I believe that overuse of the untrained muscles of the
back in jobs — be they domestic or occupational — results in
similar cramps, causing acute back pain or, in some instances,
chronic backache.

These cramps readily simulate other traumatic conditions of
the joints of the back and are mistakenly diagnosed as such.
In the summer months the rapid recovery from symptoms of
acute back pain in patients such as I have described, especially
without any specific treatment, can only be ascribed to some
such situation. Cardiac patients on salt free diets complain of
odd aches and discomforts during the hot weather and they are
limited in activity. This clinical observation would lend support
to my contention. At least it would cause no material hardship
to industry, the armed forces, employers of unskilled laborers
and do-it-yourself fans to insist on adequate fluid intake and the
ingestion of supplementary salt during the summer months as
an attempt at prophylaxis against disability from episodes of
acute back pain. There is a wide field for research in the part
played by water and electrolyte imbalance in the production of

pain of muscle origin, and, for that matter, in osteoarthritis and other "arthritic" diseases.

Panniculo-fibrositis. There is one other form of fibrositis found in the back which accompanies any loss of joint movement from whatever cause. This is manifested by the adherence of the skin and superficial fascia to the deep fascia, and even through the interstitial tissue throughout the muscles. It is detected by skin rolling directly over the spine (see page 74), and, when diffuse fibrositis is present, over these areas also. It is not peculiar to the back because it is also found over a pathologically tight iliotibial band. I call this diffuse panniculo-fibrositis and its importance is that it can cause joint dysfunction in the back if untreated. It is, however, normally secondary to joint dysfunction.

Symptoms of Fibrositis. The symptoms and signs of fibrositis in the back may be confusing and bizarre and the treatment of the condition anything but straightforward.

The symptoms are pain, either local or diffuse, in the soft tissues. The pain may be acute and knifelike, or chronic and aching. It may migrate from place to place. For signs, there may be tender nodules fairly easily localized and palpated or there may be just diffuse pain on skin rolling. There may be local or diffuse muscle spasm and resultant apparent loss of joint movement. There is increased stiffness with rest, which is more marked if an infective element is present. The symptoms and signs may be sufficiently severe to produce diagnostic confusion to the extent of suspecting conditions such as acute anterior poliomyelitis or serious bone or joint disease as being the cause of them. These patients may even run a mild pyrexia. On the other hand, the symptoms and signs may be so indefinite that the patient is labeled a hypochondriac, neurotic, hysteric or, sometimes even, a malingerer.

Treatment. Treatment (not just palliation) of fibrositis to be successful must start by removal of the cause. Sometimes this is sufficient in itself to cure the fibrositis attack.

The application of heat and gentle pétrissage (kneading massage) will usually be sufficient to relieve the symptoms of cold fibrositis.

The diffuse form of fibrositis is best treated by hot moist air baths, followed by pétrissage, and finishing each treatment with light effleurage. In the moist air bath, it is sufficient if the oral temperature rises to 100° F., or at the most 101° F. It is interesting that the sweat of the patient in this bath is strongly acid to litmus paper at the start of treatment, and at the end of about 20 minutes becomes more neutral. This acid reaction of the sweat becomes less and less marked as the patient's condition improves.

More localized tender areas may respond simply to spraying the skin over the area with ethyl chloride, followed by deep friction massage; or infiltration with local anesthetic may be required. In resistant cases, other more special forms of physical therapy may be indicated. In these patients, attention to diet, anemia, and other deviations from normal health is important. Salicylates or iodides by mouth also seem to help many of them.

The condition referred to as panniculo-fibrositis can only be treated by the special form of massage which is called skin rolling. This is performed in the same manner as described for diagnostic skin rolling on page 74. Sometimes the back is too tender to allow manual skin rolling to be performed. Then cupping massage has to be used first. It seems to be impossible to obtain suction cups these days but a breast pump does well enough. The back is smeared over with vaseline and, the skin having been raised up into the cup by suction, the cup is rhythmically moved up and down over the back until a slight skin erythema is produced. The degree of suction can be controlled by the hand holding the suction bulb. The cup should not be pushed down onto the back during treatment, but rather slightly pulled away from it. Cupping should follow infrared heat; skin rolling is best done under the infrared lamp. Effleurage must complete each therapy session. When the muscles and fascia become free of pain, treatment aimed at restoring normal muscle tone must be instituted. This consists of heavy pétrissage, tapotement (beating) and active exercise. But, again, all therapy sessions should end with effleurage for relaxation and a rest period.

The use of ultrasound in combination with a surging low voltage current, following heat, combines the three therapeutic actions which are advocated — namely: (1) the production of physiological pumping action of the muscle; (2) softening areas of scar tissue, be they macro- or microscopic; and (3) diffusing collections of fluid in locally stagnant areas.

The machine which combines these therapy modalities is relatively new and expensive. When it is more readily available, the local treatment of the foregoing conditions may be more efficient. However, the basic rules of treatment remain unaltered.

The Taut Iliotibial Band

Symptoms associated with the taut iliotibial band may be just those which are normally associated with acute or chronic subluxation of one or both sacroiliac joints. When the iliotibial band is pathologically tight, however, there is a history of frequent recurrences of acute episodes of pain following insignificant trauma. The pain may be localized to the classic area medial to the posterior superior iliac spine, with or without radiation into the groin or down the front, side or back of the thigh to the knee. Pain may be present in either iliac fossa, suggesting visceral disease. Most of these symptoms in fact arise in the sacroiliac joint, but the cause of the joint subluxation being maintained (or frequently recurring) is in the iliotibial band. Symptoms may also arise from the band itself and consist of pain referred to the hip or knee or both. If the band is riddled with sensitive fibrositic deposits, as it sometimes is, then there may be a generalized aching in thigh as well. When the band becomes singularly taut, the symptoms are of a "snapping hip" as well.

The signs of a pathologically tight iliotibial band are those of subluxation, usually backward, of one sacroiliac joint together with the signs of tightness with or without tenderness which are discussed in Chapter 5. The techniques for eliciting them are illustrated in Figures 21 to 25 (pages 70–73). There is an additional sign of tightness which may be elicited. With the patient relaxed and lying on his side, the upper leg lying slightly flexed in front of the under leg (which is also slightly flexed), the iliotibial band of the upper leg is rolled backward over the greater trochanter by the examiner using the thumbs of both hands. With a normal iliotibial band, the foot of that leg simply raises at the heel and slightly internally rotates. With a tight band the whole lower leg may be raised up into the air by the maneuver.

Treatment. Treatment for this condition is twofold. First, the band must be stretched; and second, normal movement must be restored to the affected sacroiliac joint. It is useless to use either modality of treatment separately.

After Frank Ober, M.D., drew attention to the condition, many surgeons simply lengthened the band surgically, and neglected the dysfunction in the sacroiliac joint. Thus, proper treatment failed and his excellent work fell into disuse. The operation alone cannot relieve the symptoms in the back.

Only an iliotibial band which is mildly taut can be stretched adequately to remove the cause of unnatural stresses on the sacroiliac joints and the joints at the lumbosacral junction. Manual stretching will fail, even in these cases, unless the patient also undertakes a specific exercise program, which he has to continue indefinitely if the benefit from treatment is to be maintained. It is useless to continue the conservative program of treatment if it fails to produce the required result in 3 weeks. Manual stretching of the band requires hard and determined work on the part of the therapist. In my experience, this treatment can be accomplished only by a male therapist, and unless he is prepared to put in this hard work then the method of treatment had better not be attempted.

Manual Treatment. For manual stretching of the iliotibial band, the patient lies in the side-lying position with the leg which is to be treated uppermost. Both legs should be comfortably flexed at the hip and knee, and the upper leg should rest in front of the lower one.

For treatment purposes, the band is divided into three parts: (1) the band distal to the greater trochanter; (2) the band overlying the greater trochanter; (3) the band and tensor fascia lata muscle proximal to the greater trochanter. The technique of treatment is different for each part.

(1) *Technique for stretching the iliotibial band distal to the greater trochanter:* First, the anterior fibers of the band are stretched; second, the posterior fibers of the band are stretched.

The manipulative movement which is used to stretch the anterior fibers of the band distal to the greater trochanter is best appreciated if the reader considers how he would try to snap a

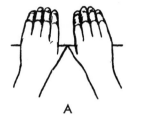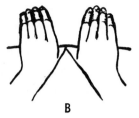

A   B

FIGURE 59. Position of hands in stretching the anterior fibers of the
iliotibial band. (A) At the beginning of the movement; (B) at the end
of the movement.

stout stick without using the knee as a fulcrum. To accomplish
this he uses his thumbs as a fulcrum on one side of the stick,
snapping the stick over the thumbs by sharply putting the fingers
through a movement of ulnar deviation away from each other.
It is in just this manner that the anterior fibers of the iliotibial
band are stretched. Figure 59 shows the position of the hands,
(A) at the beginning and (B) at the end of the movement.
Most of the breaking or stretching force is transmitted through
the proximal phalanges of the fifth fingers. The thumbs must
not pinch the band or press it up against the femur, or the procedure will be painful and unavailing. It is usual to start the
stretching at the knee and work up to the trochanter. Figure 60
shows the position adopted in this part of the treatment.

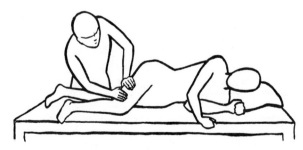

FIGURE 60. Position of hands in stretching the anterior fibers of the
iliotibial band.

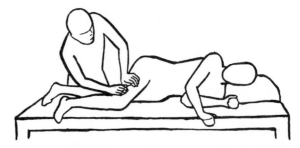

Figure 61.   Position of hands in stretching the posterior fibers of the
iliotibial band. The left hand is pushing forward, while the right hand
is stabilizing the band. The movements of the hands are then reversed.

The posterior fibers of the iliotibial band distal to the greater
trochanter are then stretched in a different manner. In this
case, the ball of each hand is used as a piston pushing against
the posterior fibers of the band, while the fingers of the other
hand stabilize the band by grasping the anterior aspect of it,
being careful not to pull it backward against the piston thrust of
the moving hand. Again the stretching starts at the knee and the
hands work stepwise up the band to the greater trochanter.
Figure 61 shows the position adopted for this part of the treatment. Figure 62 shows the common fault when using this tech-

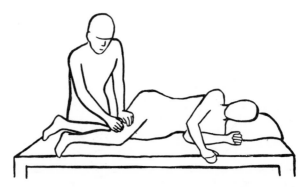

Figure 62.   Faulty technique in stretching the iliotibial band. The pressure is inserted obliquely on the back of the band and downward onto
the femur.

nique, namely, pushing the band into the femur, which bruises the band and prevents further treatment because of pain.

(2) *Technique for stretching the iliotibial band over the greater trochanter:* Figure 63 shows the leg in the position in which the stretching treatment of the iliotibial band is carried out. To stretch this small area of the iliotibial band, it is rolled backward and forward over the greater trochanter. To roll the band over the trochanter backward, the thumbs are placed on the band over the anterior aspect of the trochanter, the palms of the hands facing backward, and the thumbs being in oppo-

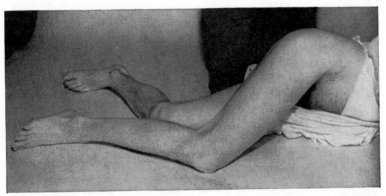

FIGURE 63.   The right leg at rest, which is the position in which the iliotibial band is stretched. The position of the right heel should be noted and compared with its position in Figure 65.

sition with their interphalangeal joints extended. Pressure is exerted through the thumbs downward onto the trochanter and backward to roll the band off the trochanter. Figure 64 illustrates the position of the mobilizing thumbs placed over the front of the trochanter prior to rolling the band backward. As the band rolls backward over the trochanter, the leg internally rotates and the heel lifts from the couch as the foot turns inward. Figure 65 shows the whole leg at the end of the stretching movement. This

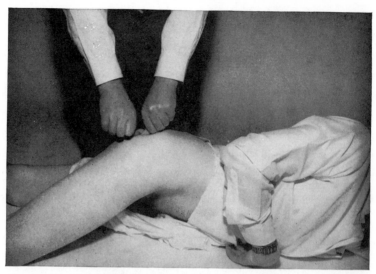

FIGURE 64.   Stretching of the iliotibial band over the greater trochanter.
Note position of the mobilizing thumbs, which are placed over the front
of the greater trochanter prior to rolling the iliotibial band backward.

illustration should be compared with Figure 63. If the heel does
not raise from the couch in the manner described (Fig. 65),
then the stretching technique is faulty.

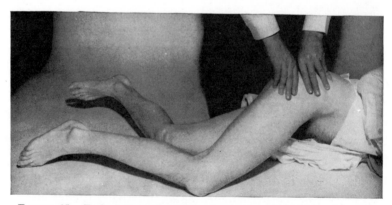

FIGURE 65.   End position adopted by the leg, the iliotibial band having
been rolled backward over the trochanter. Note the raising of the heel
on the side being treated. If the heel does not move in this manner, the
stretching technique is faulty.

To roll the band forward over the trochanter, the tips of the middle three fingers are placed on the band over the posterior aspect of the trochanter, the palms of the hands facing backward. Pressure is exerted through the finger tips downward onto the trochanter and forward to roll the band off the trochanter. Figure 66 shows the position of the hands at the end of this movement.

(3) *Technique for stretching the iliotibial band above the*

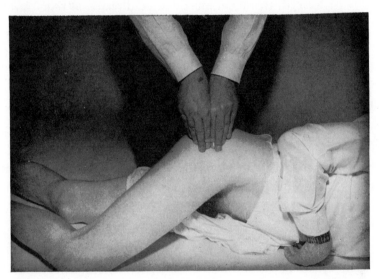

FIGURE 66.   Stretching of the iliotibial band over the greater trochanter. In this instance the iliotibial band has been rolled forward.

trochanter: The iliotibial band between the greater trochanter and the iliac crest largely consists of the tensor fascia lata muscle. Muscle, of course, cannot be stretched in the same way as the fibroelastic band. When the band is tight and tender, however, this muscle will be in spasm. This part of the band, therefore, is treated by the use of gentle kneading massage and effleurage.

There are times when the iliotibial band is too tender to start manual stretching. In these cases the diagnosis of acute diffuse fibrositis of the band is often made; but the usual treatment which may be expected to relieve this painful condition fails. This is because the tenderness in the band is due to diffuse fibrosis rather than diffuse fibrositis, and the pain arises from pulling on contracted scar tissue, the pain being aggravated by the usual forms of physical therapy which are used in the treatment of fibrositis.

When the band is too tender to allow stretching techniques to be performed, treatment must first be directed at relief of the pain. The inflammatory reaction in the band may be caused by a distant focus of infection. When such a focus is present, it must be eradicated before any other treatment is instituted. Local treatment to get rid of the tenderness in the band so that stretching may be undertaken should consist of some form of superficial heat, followed by skin rolling or cupping, followed in turn by effleurage along its length, starting at the knee and working centripetally. Superficial heat followed by ultrasound may be sufficient. In resistant cases, subcutaneous injection of oxygen is one of the most efficient means of treating very painful bands.

Renewed resilience in a previously taut band must be maintained by using the following exercises, or resilience will be rapidly lost again.

Exercise Programs. The first exercise used to stretch the right iliotibial band is as follows:

The patient stands and places the heel of the right foot into the hollow of the left foot. The right foot is then advanced half a step forward and slightly laterally and the weight of the body is transferred immediately over the advanced right foot, which is externally rotated about 30 degrees. The right knee is braced, and this rotates the femur through about 30 degrees also.

This places the greater trochanter immediately beneath the central part of the iliotibial band. Now if the leg is thrown into adduction, the band is stretched over the trochanter. Adduction of the leg is achieved by carrying the pelvis to the right without tilting it. To avoid tilting the pelvis, the left knee is allowed to bend in the same sort of way as it does when performing the follow-through of a golf stroke. Then the patient returns to the starting position. Figure 67A shows the starting position and Figure 67B illustrates the position at the end of the stretching movement with the right leg in adduction, the left knee bent and the pelvis carried over the braced right leg, the pelvis still being in the horizontal plane. The common faults in performing this exercise, vitiating its usefulness, are allowing the pelvis to tilt downward on the left, dropping the left shoulder and extending the right hip instead of adducting it. To be of any use this exercise must be performed many, many times a day.

The second exercise used to stretch the iliotibial band is as follows:

The patient stands and places himself at arm's length from

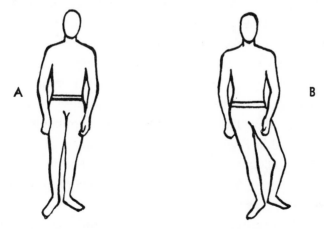

FIGURE 67. Exercise to stretch iliotibial band. (A) Starting position; (B) end position. Note that the pelvis has remained horizontal.

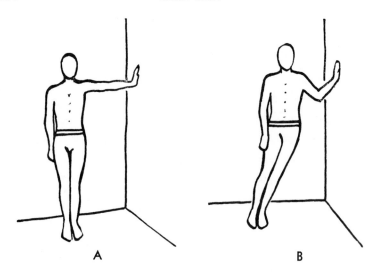

FIGURE 68. Second exercise to stretch the iliotibial band. (A) Starting position; (B) end position. Note that the pelvis remains horizontal.

a wall. The palm of his left hand, if the left iliotibial band is to be stretched, is placed flat against the wall. Figure 68A shows the starting position. The outstretched arm is now flexed at the elbow, allowing the body to approach the wall; this brings the left leg into adduction and, providing the pelvis remains horizontal, stretches the iliotibial band over the greater trochanter. Figure 68B shows the end position of this exercise. In performing this movement, the body must remain upright, and a guide to this is to be sure that the shirt buttons remain vertical with the floor. This exercise, to be of any use, must also be performed many times a day. The common faults in performing this exercise are illustrated in Figure 69; it is obvious that there is no stretch being imparted to the band in Figure 69A, and in the position adopted in Figure 69B the stretch stress is being thrown onto the lumbar spine and its supporting structures.

To stretch the opposite iliotibial band, using the exercises described, the technique and stance are simply reversed.

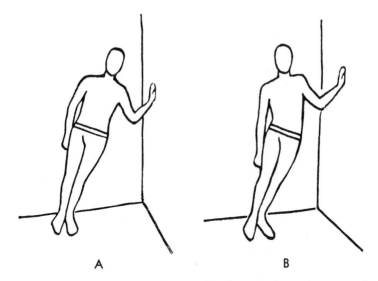

A   B

FIGURE 69.   Common faults when performing second exercise to stretch
the iliotibial band (Fig. 68). (A) The pelvis is tilted; (B) the pelvis is
tilted and the patient's movements are mainly side bending of the lumbar
spine.

Stretching the iliotibial bands is usually just a part of the
treatment of chronic dysfunction in one or both of the sacroiliac
joints—sometimes associated with dysfunction at the lumbosacral joint as well. Treatment will fail to obtain the expected
relief of symptoms unless the dysfunction in the joints is relieved
by manipulative therapy. Also, Ober's syndrome is often associated with tendo Achillis insufficiency, and treatment will also
probably fail if this insufficiency, if it is present, is not compen-
sated for by attention to the heel height of the patient's footwear.

Operative Treatment. When the band is very tight and tender,
it is a waste of time to consider any treatment short of open
tenotomy. The operation is performed with the patient in the side-
lying position. The knee of the upper leg rests on the operating
table in front of the lower leg; both legs are mildly flexed. The incision is at right angles to the band, 3 to 4 inches in length, and

lies on the lateral aspect of the thigh midway between the anterior superior iliac spine and the upper limit of the greater trochanter of the femur. The incision is carried down to the band, which can be easily recognized. The band is cut across in the line of the incision and each free end snaps away up and down the leg in a most dramatic manner. A gauze-covered, gloved finger is inserted in the wound and any part of the band still adherent to the underlying muscle is stripped away. Any tight fibrous tissue or intermuscular septa are cut. Hemostasis must be meticulous. The wound is closed in two layers by suitable interrupted sutures. A Penrose drain should be left in, since even with seemingly perfect hemostasis there is usually a large amount of oozing from the wound. Half of the drain is removed on the first postoperative day and the rest on the second postoperative day. After the wound is dressed and while the patient is still on the operating table, the patient is ready and in position for manipulation of the sacroiliac joint by the method illustrated in Figure 24, page 72. The patient is then turned on his back and the joints of the lumbosacral junction are put through their normal range of movement, using the technique illustrated in Figure 20, page 69. The patient is then returned to bed, being placed on his back with the knees flexed.

Each day this movement of the lumbosacral joints is maintained by gently side bending the pelvis, with the knees and hips flexed at right angles. Sacroiliac joint movement must be maintained, with the patient in the appropriate side-lying position, by rocking the ilium back and forth in a manner similar to that in which the manipulation was performed. On the second day the head of the bed may be rolled up to 45 degrees for meals, but the knees must be kept flexed. On the third day the patient sits on the edge of the bed with the legs dangling and may be stood up in laced Oxford walking shoes for a few moments, once or twice. On the fourth day the patient may take a few steps around the room and he is usually ready for discharge on the fifth or sixth postoperative day. The patient must never stand or walk except in his walking shoes. Postoperative physical treatment starts on the third postoperative day and is prescribed according to the secondary soft tissue problems that may have been found coexisting at the time of examination and along the lines already described. Certainly muscle re-education is essential.

The taut iliotibial band condition may be bilateral. If it is, treatment will fail unless both bands are stretched or sectioned. It is a mean thing to operate on both sides at the same time; also, early movement in bed is almost impossible when the patient has two painful surgical wounds, one on each side.

Insufficiency of the Achilles Tendons

Almost always there is insufficiency of the Achilles tendons associated with taut iliotibial bands, and that is why it has been stressed above that the patient must always wear walking shoes with heels once standing and ambulation are resumed after surgery. However, the condition may exist alone and if uncorrected prevents the success of otherwise suitable treatment of low back pain.

Treatment. Attention to the heel height of footwear is an integral part of treatment of any cause of pain in the low back. The method of assessing this insufficiency is discussed on pages 63–64, and the measurement of heel height required to compensate for it is illustrated in Figures 18 and 19 (pages 64–65). The part that adequate heels on footwear play in the postsurgical and postmanipulative treatment of back pain cannot be too greatly stressed.

"Kissing Spines"

The symptoms which arise from the so-called "kissing spines" arise from traumatic adventitious bursitis. They usually occur only in the low back and only when it is subjected to abnormal extension or hypertension. There occurs a virtual pseudar-throsis between the adjacent surfaces of two spinous processes at their posterior extremes; indeed sclerosis of the adjacent bone margins may be seen radiologically (Fig. 70). The spinous processes involved may be otherwise normal or one of them may

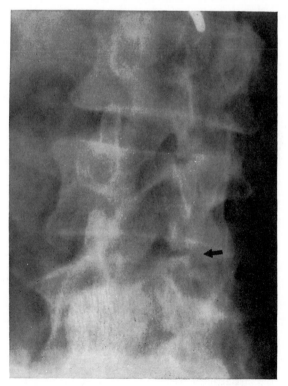

FIGURE 70. "Kissing spines" between two lumbar vertebrae. The sclerosis of the adjacent spinous process tips is apparent.

be anomalous because of, for instance, a congenital spina bifida occulta. Pain is very severe but tends to be intermittent. Subjectively it may seem to have a wide distribution, but objectively tenderness is elicited at a point well localized between the two spinous processes. Extension of the back is very limited and produces marked aggravation of the pain.

Treatment. Treatment by injection of the local area with Novocain, with or without hydrocortisone, brings immediate relief which often is lasting provided the patient is instructed not to lean over backward. A light brace, belt or corset to be worn as a conscience to remind the patient not to extend the back is sometimes necessary. In severe unremitting cases surgical removal of one of the offending spinous processes must be undertaken and is curative.

Lumbarization; Sacralization

These congenital anomalies may be considered together. Lumbarization means that the first sacral segment has the characteristics of a lumbar vertebra. Sacralization means that the fifth lumbar vertebra has the characteristics of the first sacral segment. The alterations of the involved vertebra in my experience are most often unilateral; it is certainly in the presence of the unilateral deformity that these conditions are likely to give rise to symptoms. There is one big difference between the two conditions from a clinical point of view. In cases of lumbarization, the patient in effect now has six lumbar vertebrae. This means that the strain-prone lumbar spine, by virtue of its abnormal length, is even more vulnerable to stress and trauma. In such backs there tends at all times to be excessive movement, which increases the chances that the patient will suffer from intervertebral joint strains and other traumatic injuries. This is most marked when the lumbarization anomaly is bilateral.

When these congenital anomalies are unilateral, symptoms may arise either from the pseudarthrosis, which is so often present on the anchored side, or from overmovement and instability, resulting in dysfunction in the joint on the unanchored side. Figure 71 demonstrates unilateral sacralization with the pseudarthrosis on the anchored side, i.e., the side which assumes the sacral characteristics. Pseudarthrosis is more commonly seen in sacralization than in lumbarization.

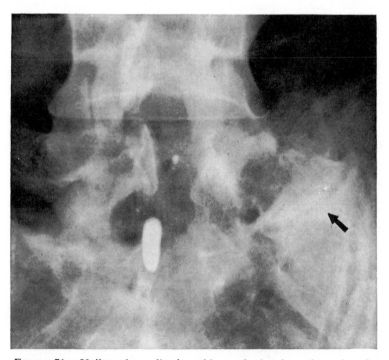

FIGURE 71. Unilateral sacralization with pseudarthrosis on the anchored side indicated by an arrow. There are advanced changes characteristic of osteoarthritis in the false joint. A laminectomy has been done on the same side. The patient's back symptoms had not been relieved by the disc surgery.

The main symptom from these conditions is low back pain, but when it arises on the anchored side the history may be very confusing. Physical signs from these conditions, too, may be very confusing, and the diagnosis may ultimately be resolved only by the X-ray picture. They can often be suspected when an unusually long sacral flattening is noted on examination and movement on bending forward seems to start higher in the low back than one would expect. The sign of pain will be elicited unilaterally, and yet not in exactly the same place that it would be found in sacroiliac joint pathology. The movements eliciting pain are those made by the patient positioning himself rather than the examining movements. The pseudarthrosis is tender to direct pressure in a place which is not one of the five classic places in relation to the posterior superior iliac spine.

Treatment. Treatment of pain arising from the pseudarthrosis consists of injection into the joint (or around the joint if entry cannot be effected) of local anesthetic, with or without hydrocortisone, and of instruction of the patient in the avoidance of unguarded twisting movements and hypertension of the low back. The injection may have to be repeated two to three times. As symptoms from the pseudarthrosis may be due to traumatic synovitis, rest may be a very necessary adjunct to therapy; also, this is a condition which may respond well to ultrasound. There are not the same contraindications to dispersing the fluid in a pseudarthrosis as there are in a normal joint in which there is synovitis.

Treatment of pain arising from the unanchored side must often be manipulative, since dysfunction is common in this anomalous unprotected interlaminar joint. Equally, the interlaminar joint may be the seat of traumatic osteoarthritis and chronic synovitis because of the constant strain and abnormal movement in the joint. Then manipulation is contraindicated, and indeed tends to worsen the joint pathology. In such a case the clue is given in the history, for there is a history of stiffness following rest rather than of relief of symptoms with rest. In this case a corset or even a back brace may be required before the patient is relieved. But whenever a back support is prescribed, muscle-strengthening exercise for the back must be prescribed too; and in this condition the importance of symmetrical exercises cannot be too highly stressed, because any twisting exercise copies a common cause of the underlying joint disability. Fusion may have to be resorted to in recalcitrant cases.

Spondylolysis; Spondylolisthesis

Symptoms from these conditions by no means arise because of the congenital laminar defect or the slipping forward of one

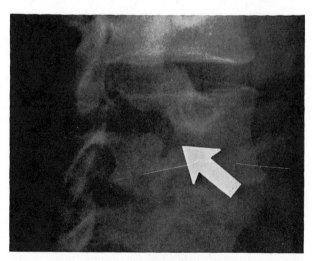

FIGURE 72. An extreme congenital laminar defect without slipping of the vertebral body. The condition was diagnosed clinically and relief of symptoms from the joints was obtained by alteration of weight bearing, remedial exercises, and manipulation.

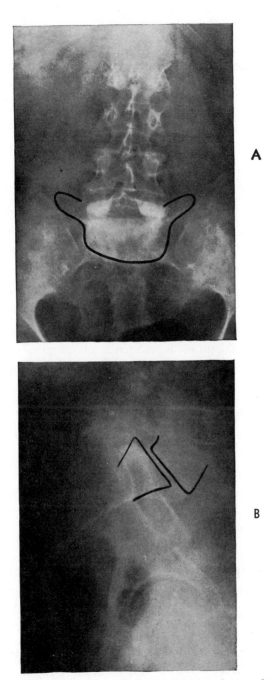

FIGURE 73. Spondylolisthesis. (A) Anteroposterior view used to show the Bow Line of Brailsford. The appearance at the lumbosacral junction should be compared with the relatively normal lumbosacral junction in Figure 76 (page 201). (B) Typical lateral view of same patient.

vertebral body on another *per se*. Not all patients with pain and spondylolisthesis need a spine fusion. Careful examination of patients who have pain with these conditions reveals many other causes of their symptom, which have been discussed, and appropriate physical treatment will relieve the patient. Figure 72 illustrates a gross laminar defect at the fourth lumbar junction in such a patient.

Many patients have anteroposterior X-ray views of their spine taken during a diagnostic work-up. The Bow Line sign of Brailsford (Fig. 73) is a helpful radiological sign of spondylolisthesis which is demonstrated in the anteroposterior projection. By this sign spondylolisthesis can be diagnosed from flat plates of the abdomen, scout films of kidney, ureter and bladder, and from films taken for barium studies of the bowel. Figure 73B shows the spondylolisthesis of the case used to illustrate Figure 73A in the usual lateral projection. Such a radiological diagnosis may give the clue to where to look for the site of a patient's symptoms which remain otherwise mysterious.

Other Conditions

There remain a few conditions which give rise to pain in the back which are not pertinent to the immediate thesis yet which may confuse the physician and can be ameliorated by suitable physical therapy.

Infective Spondylitis. The pain of infective spondylitis from acute prostatitis or pelvic inflammatory disease is rapidly relieved by pelvic diathermy.

Ankylosing Spondylitis. The intractable pain of ankylosing spondylitis, which may persist even after X-ray therapy, can be ameliorated by spinal subtonal faradism. By subtonal faradism is meant the use of the faradic current of constant intensity (heretofore reference to faradism has been concerned with surging of the current) between two stationary electrodes placed at either end of the spine. The intensity of the current should be that which just does not cause muscle contraction. (See also Chapter 12.)

Osteoporosis Senilis. The pain associated with osteoporosis senilis seems more rapidly to be relieved if the patient is given tonic courses of ultraviolet light in addition to the usual treatment of Albright's regime and exercise.

Postural Joint Strain. Pain from postural joint strain which does not arise from diagnosable joint dysfunction may be relieved by remedial exercises. Redistribution of weight bearing may have to be obtained by adjusting the heel height of the patient's footwear before permanent relief can be obtained. Any well-trained therapist can teach suitable remedial exercises, which need not, therefore, be detailed here.

Sacral Pain. Sacral pain is sometimes confusing diagnostically. There are but few local causes of sacral pain of which I am aware. Usually it is referred from the viscera within the pelvis. The commonest exceptions are the presence of periosteal bruising, a fissure fracture following direct trauma, or chordoma of the sacrum. Periosteal bruising can be treated by counter irritation either using contact ultraviolet light, employing the third erythema plus dose every fourth day for three or four applications, or using a reactive dose of histamine ionization, employing a disc anode as the active electrode. Sometimes infiltration of a local anesthetic is sufficient.

Asthma. A word about the use of manipulative therapy in the treatment of asthma is not out of place. Spinal manipulation never cured asthma. It may abort an attack of asthma and it may relieve the intensity of an asthmatic attack; and the relief obtained from either of these may be sufficient for the patient to claim that manipulation has produced a cure. The reason for the relief which the asthmatic obtains from manipulation of the thoracic spine and costovertebral joints should be obvious. In an asthmatic attack, the auxiliary muscles of respiration go into spasm in inspiration when the patient cannot exhale. One of the common causes of joint dysfunction is unrelieved muscle spasm. The small normal excursion of each individual costovertebral joint is easily lost with intercostal muscle spasm. Further, the interlaminar joints of the thoracic spine are splinted in the asthmatic by the back muscles, and the poor normal movement of an asthmatic's chest never allows their full range of movement to take place. Pain from one of these joints in which there is dysfunction may precipitate an asthmatic attack and maintenance of joint function may lessen the frequency of, or abort, an attack. The maintenance of normal joint function makes it easier for an asthmatic to breathe and the attacks may be less frequent or less severe when they do occur.

No program of physical therapy should last longer than 4 weeks at the most when treating back pain. It should not last longer than a week in the absence of definite improvement in both the patient's symptoms *and* signs. If the patient does not show such improvement, either subjectively or objectively, the wrong diagnosis has been made and/or the wrong treatment has been prescribed.

11

The Intervertebral Disc and Back Pain

Almost no mention of the intervertebral disc has been made in its relation to back pain. This is for two reasons: first, I do not believe that manipulative treatment has any part in the primary treatment of disc lesions; and second, it is my belief that the intervertebral disc does not usually play primarily a large part in the production of symptoms of pain in the back, with or without radiating pain in the extremities.

I realize that this belief flies in the face of the present trend, but this is one of the major reasons why I believe pain from the back is currently being unsatisfactorily handled.

In support of this belief is the fact that there is one small segment of the spine in which there are no intervertebral discs. Yet a patient who suffers from traumatic pathology in this area presents symptoms of pain, both local to the joints in the area and radiating along the segmental nerves, that occur in just the same manner and with just the same intensity as the symptoms of pain produced by similar trauma at levels where there are discs.

The area of the spine without discs is, of course, at the junctions between the occiput and the atlas and between the atlas and the axis. Trauma is frequently inflicted at these two intervertebral levels. When these joints are injured, the patient as frequently complains of local pain with radiation up into the head along the segmental nerves — the greater and lesser occipital and the greater auricular nerves — as he complains of pain, both local and radiating, when the low back is injured. Symptoms from trauma in the thoracic spine, namely, local pain radiating around the chest or into the abdomen, and symptoms from trauma in the cervical spine, namely, local pain radiating into the arms, are analogous.

The common anatomy in all these areas is the synovial joints, of which there are one hundred thirty-five from the occiput to the sacrum (including the sacroiliac joints, costovertebral joints, and joints of Luschka), whereas there are only twenty-three discs. The joints of Luschka are probably synovial, but their relation to pain symptoms must be highly conjectural.

The fact that pathology in synovial joints does give rise to distant referred symptoms of pain is well recognized, and the classic example of this is that the presenting symptom of hip pathology is frequently pain felt in the knee. If pathology in the joints of the extremities can produce referred pain, it is logical to postulate that joints, similar in every anatomical and physiological feature, in the back behave in the same way when subjected to the same pathology.

Of course there can be no disagreement with the fact that an intervertebral disc may primarily give rise to back pain, with or without radiation. But I believe that the prolapse of the nucleus pulposus is a rare cause of these symptoms, and that when it does occur, the symptoms and signs are clear and the treatment by enucleation of the disc is certain.

I think a great deal of confusion in the treatment of back conditions would be dispelled if we ceased to talk about "discs" and "disc lesions." When a nucleus pulposus prolapses, it becomes an epidural tumor, using the word tumor in its broadest sense — "a swollen or distended part . . . possessing no physio-logical function" (*Webster's New Collegiate Dictionary*, 1953). The signs of a space-occupying tumor are those of pressure on the anatomical structures which belong in that space, and which are being displaced by that which does not belong there. Further, the treatment of a tumor producing symptoms is perfectly clear, namely, its enucleation. I also believe that the conservative treat-ment of a prolapsed disc is its surgical removal, just as the con-servative treatment of acute appendicitis is the removal of the appendix.

Diagnosis of Disc Lesions

Prolapse. I do not consider that the diagnosis of a "disc lesion" should be made unless the majority of the following items of examination are positive:

(1) There must be, at some time in the history of the patient's complaint, an accident of sufficient severity to injure the annulus fibrosus and to weaken it by scar formation.

(2) There must be a subsequent injury, by history, of suffi-cient severity to rupture the weakened annulus fibrosus and to allow prolapse of the nucleus pulposus. Remembering that inter-vertebral discs degenerate because of toxic factors, or, pre-sumably, because of repetitive minor trauma, maybe a single injury will precipitate the prolapse. The classic example of disc degeneration from toxic factors used to be seen in cases of typhoid fever. I am now of the opinion that deficient nutrition of a patient may play a significant part in disc degeneration.

(3) At some prior time to the present illness, the patient must have complained of pain in the back.

(4) On examination there must be clinical evidence in the spine of mechanical derangement of a segmental nature in the region of the prolapsed disc. This mechanical derangement from

the joint lock of the neighboring joints causes dysfunction in them.

(5) There must be mixed neurological signs, i.e., objective signs of motor and sensory defect. It is most unlikely that pressure on a nerve root would only pick out either sensory or motor fibers, even though the sensory fibers are said to be located peripherally in the nerves. An early motor sign of a low lumbar disc prolapse is the atrophy of the extensor brevis digitorum muscle of the foot. If the prolapse is central rather than lateral, one would not expect radicular signs. In such cases, which are rare, the pain symptom probably arises from the dura. In assessing neurological signs in the legs, it is essential to interpret the straight-leg-raising sign correctly (the reader is referred to comments on this subject to be found in the section dealing with the examination of the low back on pages 66 to 68).

(6) The protein in the spinal fluid should be raised. It is classic of thecal irritation that the protein content of the spinal fluid is raised both above and below an irritative lesion. A truly lateral prolapse may not irritate the theca, but in such a situation the objective radicular signs should be very clear. I have found an elevated protein on the third day following the initial onset of acute back symptoms from a prolapsed disc.

(7) In doubtful cases in the lumbar spine, the performance of an epidural injection may be diagnostic. A disc prolapse is only doubtful in diagnosis in the spine in the low lumbar region, i.e., below the third lumbar vertebra, as this is the only area where there is room for an epidural tumor to be present without giving clear pressure signs. In the average person, it should be possible to inject 100 cc. of fluid into the epidural space through the sacrococcygeal hiatus without any discomfort to the patient. This amount of fluid reaches up to the third lumbar vertebra in the average spine. If there is an epidural mass or block, as soon

as the fluid hits it, the patient experiences acute pain from pressure on it. The pain is an exacerbation of the patient's symptom pain. The advantage of this procedure is that it may be curative if the condition which is present is a true sciatic neuritis. For the injection, one uses from 10 to 20 cc. of 2 per cent procaine, followed by up to 80 to 90 cc. of 2 per cent saline. If a sciatic nerve root is edematous, the edema fluid is presumably withdrawn from the nerve root into the hypertonic injection fluid by osmosis; relief of symptoms in such a case is not only instantaneous, but also very dramatic.

(8) X-rays. The diagnosis of a disc prolapse as the primary cause of symptoms can never be made from the appearance of the disc space in plain X-ray films, any more than the presence of spondylolisthesis detected by X-rays means that this is the cause of symptoms. The diminution of a disc space is by no means pathognomonic of a prolapsed disc. The appearance of osteophytes around the periphery of a vertebral body is suggestive of disc degeneration and bulging of the disc beyond its normal confines, but practically never is such osteophytic formation found posteriorly on the vertebral bodies; and so this condition is in no way pathognomonic of a prolapse. These bony changes and their significance are discussed in a subsequent section (see page 197).

(9) Myelogram and Discogram. To complete this syndrome of signs of disc prolapse, consideration must be given to the myelogram and discogram, even though I do not consider them to be necessary to arrive at the correct diagnosis. Certainly in doubtful cases, they may confirm a diagnosis; the pathology can be accurately diagnosed when the discogram is used, but is still indefinite when the myelogram is used. In the average case, however, their use adds unnecessary expense to the patient and risks unnecessary morbidity. I believe that, by the use of the clinical

examination earlier described and the careful consideration of the first seven criteria of diagnosis in this section, an accurate diagnosis of the presence of space-occupying pathology and its level can be made, and will justify surgical exploration. Clinical determination of the level is made by the signs elicited, especially by the two examining procedures, skin rolling and direct pressure over the individual vertebrae. If maximum tightness and tenderness on skin rolling coincides with maximum pain on direct pressure over a vertebra, then the disc involved is the one immediately below this vertebra.

Neurological signs, though often unreliable, may help in the clinical determination of the level, especially in the low lumbar spine where almost constantly a prolapse of the fourth lumbar disc involves the fifth lumbar nerve, and a prolapse of the fifth lumbar disc involves the first sacral nerve.

Certainly a myelographic defect is very characteristic of a prolapsed disc, but it is also characteristic of spinal cord or cauda equina tumors, hemangiomata, or even an epidural abscess, or hypertrophied ligamentum subflavum. But supposing there are multiple myelographic defects? This certainly does not help to determine the level from which the symptoms are arising. Further, even in the most practiced hands, the myelogram is, by common consent, 40 per cent inaccurate either by showing a defect for which no cause can be found at surgery, or by failing to show a defect in the presence of a prolapsed disc.

The discogram, however, is perfectly accurate in demonstrating a disc prolapse in that the injected contrast medium can be seen escaping into the epidural space. But the protagonists of discography usually advocate the exploration of at least three discs by this method, because clinically they are in doubt as to the level at which they expect to find the pathology. Thus a normal disc may be injected with the contrast medium, and I have seen a syringe broken by the great pressure required to introduce the fluid into a normal disc. To introduce a noxious fluid into a normal physiological disc under such pressure surely may produce the initial trauma to it to which reference is made in item (1) (see page 179) of the syndrome outlined above. And this may be the precipitating factor of degeneration, and later prolapse of this disc, which might otherwise have remained normal.

Some people claim that discography may be therapeutic if hydrocortisone is added to the injected contrast medium. In my own experience of this technique, the only patients who experienced temporary relief of their symptoms were the ones who had a frank rupture of the annulus fibrosus. Presumably their relief came from the escape of the hydrocortisone into the epidural space, where its anti-inflammatory properties were able to act directly on the nerve roots, or the hypertonic fluid acted, as it is suggested it does, when the epidural injection is performed. I can see no advantage to this over the epidural injection discussed in item 7 (see page 180) of this syndrome; and there are several disadvantages.

The additional exposure of the patient to X-radiation in performing these procedures makes their routine use unjustified.

Disc Degeneration. There are two other ways in which a disc may play a secondary role in the production of symptoms in the back. When a disc degenerates, it loses its space-occupying mass. Just like any other piece of mechanical construction, when a washer wears out, the parts which are being held by the washer in a certain spatial relationship lose that relationship and are able to move either through a greater range or a less specific range of movement than normal, becoming unstable. Thus the interlaminar synovial joints are subjected to abnormal move-

ment, their supporting ligaments become lax, and any unguarded movement to which they may be subjected may precipitate locking of the joints and dysfunction. Further, the
articular cartilages become traumatized and changes of traumatic
arthritis begin to occur; then doubtless, there follow intermittent
episodes of synovitis within the joint capsules. Under such conditions, there is little to be gained by directing treatment at the
disc. Treatment must be directed at the joints to maintain their
normal movement, and at their supporting muscles to compensate for the laxity of their supporting ligaments. Correction of
weight bearing and posture again play an important role in
prophylaxis against recurrent joint strain and joint dysfunction.

If the relationship is studied between the interlaminar joints
and the nerve roots as the latter pass out through their foramina
over the pedicles, and, in the lumbar region, where the posterior
divisions of the nerves pass between the mammillary and acces-
sory processes, it will be seen that this relationship of the nerves
to the joints is as intimate (if not more intimate) as the relationship of these nerve roots to the posterior aspects of the intervertebral discs. It is not difficult to visualize that pressure may be
exerted on these nerves by a capsule distended by synovial fluid
(or even by blood) following trauma, giving rise to signs of neuritis, neuronitis or radiculitis. These signs resolve as the swelling of
the joint subsides; this to me is the only possible explanation
of the cures achieved in so-called disc lesions treated alone by
rest and traction. But in these cases I believe that the diagnosis
of a disc lesion is erroneous. Certainly the treatment prescribed
is that which is commonly prescribed for acute synovitis in the
joints of the extremities. It is beyond my powers of imagination
to believe that a prolapsed nucleus can ever slip back within a
ruptured annulus pulposus, let alone as a result of rest and
traction.

Compressed Disc. The other injury in which a disc may play a part in producing pain — though I must admit it is speculative — is when the disc is suddenly and directly compressed, severely altering its hydrodynamics, if only momentarily. This forces the laminar articular facets into one another, creating a single acute traumatic episode, producing acute traumatic arthritis. When a similar injury is sustained by a joint of an extremity, the patient suffers from a very singular pain unlike other joint pains. These acute traumatic episodes resolve with rest in a very short period. I think this happens in the back.

Treatment

In advocating surgery as the conservative treatment for a prolapsed disc, I realize that many surgeons are reluctant to perform surgery for this condition: first, because the results of disc surgery are anything but uniformly successful in that the patient is so often left with residual back pain; and second, because the diagnosis in many surgeons' minds remains doubtful, and surgery is recommended only as a rather radical last resort. I cannot subscribe to the doubt which haunts people in diagnosis. By careful history taking and good clinical examination, the diagnosis readily becomes apparent.

Traction. In a case of very acute back pain, in which a good clinical examination cannot be undertaken at once, a short period of bed rest should be prescribed, using either pelvic traction in cases in which the low back is involved, or head traction in cases in which the neck is involved. The most satisfactory method of pelvic traction is illustrated in Figure 74, the pull of the traction producing not only a pull in the long axis

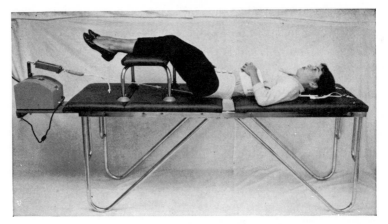

FIGURE 74. Pelvic traction; for efficient traction the hips and knees must be flexed to flatten the lumbar spine. (Courtesy of Tru-Eze Manufacturing Company.)

but also a pelvic tilt in flexion. Traction, using this apparatus, can be steady or intermittent, the latter being indicated if the underlying pathology is primarily synovitis. As in the cervical spine, efficient traction can only be obtained in the low back if the lordosis is flattened. This is achieved by flexing the hips and knees. Leg traction has little to recommend it, and very adequate work has been done to show that 10 pounds of leg traction on each leg produces no appreciable pull at the lumbosacral junction, or anywhere in the lumbar spine. Leg traction is so uncomfortable if the patient tries to move that its chief effect would seem to be to keep him immobile. It has been suggested earlier that immobility in itself is a cause of back pain, so that even this property of leg traction is undesirable.

With regard to head traction, it is often more effective when applied in the sitting rather than in the lying position. It must be remembered that to be efficient at all, cervical traction must be applied through the occiput, and not the chin. The cervical lordosis must be flattened before the intervertebral junctions can

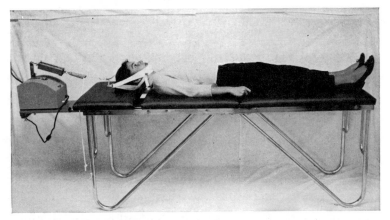

FIGURE 75. Cervical traction. The cervical spine is flattened by dropping the chin onto the neck, thereby ensuring efficiency as most of the
pull of the traction must come from the occiput with the cervical lordosis
flattened. (Courtesy of Tru-Eze Manufacturing Company.)

be distracted. Figure 75 illustrates neck traction correctly applied in the prone position.

A very satisfactory way to produce rest in the lumbar spine,
and without immobilizing the patient, is by use of the flexion
plaster jacket.

Having obtained relaxation of a patient suffering from one
of these acute episodes by the use of one of the methods suggested, it is then possible to carry out an adequate diagnostic
examination. It should never take longer than 10 days at the
most for the patient to become sufficiently relaxed for the physician to accomplish this. Very often it can be done within 2 or
3 days.

Surgery. First, the causes of the failure of surgery must be considered.

The first cause of failure, obviously, is that the preoperative
diagnosis may be erroneous. This problem should become less

and less prevalent as better clinical assessment of a patient is adopted.

The second reason for surgical failures is the fact that the operation for removal of the disc is expected to relieve not only the cause of the radicular or dural symptoms, but presumably also to correct all the mechanical derangement which is commonly accepted as being diagnostic of the "disc lesion." How the removal of disc material lying free in the epidural space, or scooped out from between the vertebral bodies, is expected to achieve this is beyond my comprehension. Certainly moving the patient to and from the operating table and positioning him on the operating table subjects him to a considerable amount of inexpert joint manipulation — sometimes very violent manipulation — both in the lumbar and cervical spines. The remarkable manipulative maneuvers to which some anesthetists subject the joints of the cervical spine during intubation have been commented upon earlier. I suspect that the mechanical spinal derangement is often overcome in some such manner in many cases in which surgery is successful in relieving both the spinal and radicular symptoms.

Lastly, one of the common reasons that surgery properly performed fails to bring expected relief is inadequate postoperative care (see page 190).

So, I believe that there would be fewer surgical failures, or partial failures, if more attention were paid to the obvious interlaminar joint and sacroiliac joint dysfunction which invariably coexists with a prolapsed disc. At the time of surgery, manipulative procedures should be undertaken to restore normal movement to the joints adjacent to the prolapse.

Spine Fusion. There is always a question of whether a spine fusion should be done at the same time as a disc enucleation.

Probably many who advocate spine fusion with disc surgery do so because they believe that the back symptoms are arising from the neighboring synovial joints, and this is the only way of being sure that the joints will no longer give rise to symptoms. Some fuse the spine empirically. Others consider that there is never any need for spine fusion, because to them obviously the disc is the pathological condition causing all the trouble.

Somewhere between these beliefs lies a happy mean. I believe that spine fusion should be done in cases where, at the time of surgery: (1) obvious overmovement or instability can be demonstrated in the joints; (2) there is a congenital anomaly present, especially that of unilateral sacralization or lumbarization; (3) there is complete lumbarization, with six vertebrae having lumbar characteristics, which produces the long sway back; (4) the fifth lumbar vertebra rides high on the sacrum, instead of snugly between the posterior superior iliac spines; (5) the facet joints at the lumbosacral junction, instead of being vertical, are what I call the universal type of joints; (6) there is spondylolisthesis or spondylolysis accompanying the disc prolapse; and (7) there is an associated crush fracture and/or vertebral dislocation.

This list of conditions which may coexist with a disc prolapse does not provide absolute indications for spine fusion. The patient's age and occupation are factors which must be taken into account. Each case must be decided on its merits.

Spine fusion also presents many problems of postsurgical management. To condemn a patient to 4 months of plaster immobilization is a formidable thing for the treatment of back pain in an otherwise healthy individual, and an uneconomical situation necessarily must arise in accepting this treatment for a family breadwinner.

I am satisfied that prolonged immobilization in plaster is unnecessary and undesirable following simple spine fusion. I have had the advantage of observing the work of Roy M. Hoover, M.D., who does a modified Hibbs type of fusion in these cases, under epidural anesthesia whenever possible.

Because he does a meticulous subperiosteal dissection of the paravertebral muscles, which, with the attached periosteum and supraspinous ligaments, can then be laid back almost perfectly over the bone grafts, he is able successfully to apply the principles of early ambulation to almost all spine fusion cases, other than cases of adolescent scoliosis and paraplegic instability. If the paravertebral muscles are damaged and torn during the dissecting process, early ambulation may lead to failure of fusion.

Postoperative Care. The postoperative program which he uses is as follows: On the day after surgery he sits the patient up on the side of the bed and the following day allows him to sit in a chair. Bathroom privileges are allowed on the day of operation if necessary to avoid catheterization or gas accumulation. From this, the patient progresses to ambulation and is able to return home in not more than 8 to 14 days. He is encouraged to walk as far and as often as possible, but he should not drive in a car for 2 months. A woman must not hang up clothes or make beds. Climbing stairs should be avoided for 2 months. Stooping activities are contraindicated for the same period of time. Return to work, other than heavy laboring, is aimed at at the end of 2 months unless he can walk to work, when work can be resumed in a month. The patient may wear a lumbosacral belt or corset after the sutures are removed for from 4 to 6 months. A corset is worn after a thoracic spine fusion. This sort of routine is not followed for cervical spine fusion because of its obvious mechanical limitations.

This is a perfectly logical way in which to manage these cases and can materially hasten recovery following simple disc surgery.

It relies on the natural support of a well-repaired lumbar fascia, together with limitation of movement at the fusion site by muscle spasm and the avoidance of stress activities. These things are more efficient than the average ill-fitting plaster spica. The patient has to be taught how to avoid movement in the fusion site when changing position from standing to sitting, and from sitting to lying, but this should not present any difficulty.

The postoperative management of a spine fusion in which the patient is returned to bed for 10 days to 3 weeks and is then put in plaster for 3 to 4 months has nothing to commend it in the average case.

Pain at the donor site, if a graft has been taken from the ilium, is readily alleviated by anodal galvanism, or by Novocain ionization, over the donor site. The use of bone wax to prevent oozing from the donor site materially lessens pain in this area.

Most of the failures of spine surgery, whether it is performed for disc or joint pathology, or, for that matter, for any neurological condition or bone disease, arise from inadequate postoperative care of the back, usually because of ignorance of methods of physical treatment: (1) to lessen pain and resulting muscle spasm; (2) to retrain muscles damaged by surgery; (3) to promote healing of muscle with minimal scarring; and (4) to maintain mobility in the joints in which there has been dysfunction.

The operating surgeon should help the patient to get out of bed initially and not delegate this duty to an assistant, nurse or therapist. The patient should move to the side of the bed, and then turn on his side to face the side of the bed. He should then flex his hips and knees to 90 degrees. Then the surgeon should assist the patient into the sitting position, being sure to keep the spine, pelvis and legs moving as a whole, and without allowing side bending to occur anywhere in the trunk. Then, before step-

ping down to the floor, the patient's walking shoes, which should
be laced shoes with adequate heels, should be put on. To reach
the floor without jarring, it may be necessary to use steps at the
side of the bed. In stepping down, the patient steadies himself,
preferably without assistance. The amount of confidence with
which the patient performs these maneuvers if the surgeon himself assists cannot be achieved by anyone else to whom the duty
of assisting is delegated. After the first time, the supervision of
a nurse or therapist is usually sufficient. The return to bed for the
first time is equally important and is carried out in the reverse
steps, again assisted by the surgeon.

The importance of having the patient wear laced, Oxford-type
walking shoes on getting up for the first time, and thereafter,
cannot be too highly stressed. From the moment the patient gets
up he should be taught to walk; he must never be allowed to
shuffle, for a shuffling gait in itself is detrimental to posture.
Shuffling in heelless bedroom slippers stretches all the soft tissues
down the back of the leg, including, of course, the sciatic nerve,
and throws a flattening strain on the lumbar lordosis. At a time
when the muscles are "soft" and the joints are lax, it can be seen
how easily a patient may perpetuate symptoms from — or even
precipitate — postural joint strain and dysfunction. Continued
stretching of the sciatic nerve perpetuates the radiculitis, or at
least delays its resolution.

The posture of the patient in bed is just as important as his
posture on resuming activity. When lying on his back, the hips
and knees should be slightly flexed. He should be encouraged to
turn from side to side frequently, but this should be done without
twisting the pelvis on the spine. Pulling on the bed rail usually
provides sufficient assistance.

Postmanipulative Care. After manipulation under anesthesia to correct dysfunction *of long standing,* particularly in the low back, a slower postoperative course is advised, to allow return of normal tonus to the muscles, which not only have been so long in spasm, but also most certainly have atrophied, and to the supporting ligaments of the joint. The patient should be rolled up into the sitting position by degrees, starting not later than 48 hours after manipulation, but as the upright position is approached, the knees must be more and more flexed. When the bed is rolled up to 45 degrees or more, a small soft pillow should be placed in the small of the back to support the lumbar lordosis. The head should not be thrust forward by a pillow behind it, though a small soft pillow may be placed behind the neck.

Erector spinae setting exercises may be started in bed 48 hours postoperatively, and faradic treatment to the muscles will shorten the period of their recovery. Both the exercises and the faradism should be undertaken within the limit of pain and gradually increased. From setting exercises, progression to assisted active exercises, done symmetrically, should be made. Any unduly painful area in the soft tissues should be treated with anodal galvanism or sedative ionization, and each treatment session should finish with a period of effleurage.

The patient should be ready to leave the hospital in an average period of 6 days. Ideally he should spend the next 3 to 4 weeks in a convalescent institution where plunge bath facilities are available. The water should be warm or hot and of a high specific gravity.

During the first week of convalescent therapy, 10 minutes of graduated back extension exercises in the bath four times a day, followed by a half to one hour rest period in bed, is the most satisfactory routine. In addition, once a day for half an hour the patient should have physical therapy as required; this may include anodal galvanism to a residually tender sciatic nerve, faradism to the back muscles, skin rolling for any associated panniculo-fibrositis, histamine ionization to any especially resistant tender area, and finally, effleurage to the back to produce relaxation.

The patient should do no walking except to and from treatments, meals, and the bathroom. When sitting in a chair, the patient is taught to keep his buttocks against the back of the seat and to sit up. When he feels tired, he should go to bed and lie down. The patient is forbidden to stoop or to lift and is taught to pick things up from the floor by squatting. He also must avoid balancing on one leg when dressing or undressing.

In the second week of convalescent care, the patient should start going for walks of no more than a quarter of a mile, the distance being increased every few days. The only other change in therapy this week is that during his physical therapy sessions he starts assisted back extension exercises in the treatment room.

In the third week, the patient progresses to unassisted back extension exercises on getting up in the morning and going to bed at night, and starts lifting weights in his therapy sessions, using his legs and not his back. Stooping from the hips is a habit of laziness which has to be broken.

At the end of the third week, the patient is usually ready to go home and should return to work a week later. If his work is heavy, he should ideally be allowed to do light duties for the next 2 to 3 months, and during this period his work should be graduated and supervised. An intelligent patient is usually able to graduate his own work satisfactorily. Stooping, twisting, and lifting with the back muscles are absolutely contraindicated. Symmetrical back extension exercises night and morning should be continued indefinitely.

Where convalescent centers are not available, the above routine is impractical, but in the suggested regime there is much that can be done in a well-designed home program.

The common practice of keeping patients in hospital without physical therapy for 2 or 3 weeks postoperatively or following manipulation and then sending them home for an indefinite period of unsupervised "rest" before returning them to their normal activities is, I am sure, a major reason for failure of surgery and joint manipulation to achieve its purpose — namely, the relief of all symptoms. Unless a consistent and intelligent effort is made to re-educate these patients, there must always be a grave risk that their disability may be as great (if not greater) as it was before surgery or manipulation.

Criticism leveled at the expense of the routine outlined above is penny wise and pound foolish. If 3 or 4 weeks of carefully regulated convalescent care can save a patient from months or years of unregulated unemployment, the economic advantage to both patient and community must be obvious.

12

The Role of Arthritis in Back Pain

The most commonly used alternative diagnosis to a disc injury as the cause of pain in the back is "arthritis." This is a slovenly term to use for diagnosis, for without a descriptive prefix, the term is meaningless.

Osteoarthritis

What is usually meant is osteoarthritis, and this diagnosis is based on the hypertrophic lipping, visualized radiographically, around the rims of the vertebral bodies.

The intellectual dishonesty of such a diagnosis is beginning to be recognized, but by no means universally. This perivertebral lipping has nothing whatever to do with osteoarthritis. Osteoarthritis is a change peculiar to synovial joints and, in the spine, can occur only in the interlaminar joints, the sacroiliac joints, the odontoatlantal joint, the costovertebral joints, and perhaps in the joints of Luschka. It can never occur in relation to the intervertebral disc joints. It is surprising how seldom the synovial joints of the spine show the changes characteristic of osteoarthritis.

Having examined the spines of some hundreds of Egyptian

196

mummies, L. R. Shore, M.D., in 1936 coined the descriptive term "polyspondylitis marginalis osteophytica" for the condition of osteophytic lipping around the vertebral bodies. He reported his work in the *British Journal of Surgery*.* He observed to me later that these osteophytic excrescences almost never were found posteriorly on the vertebral bodies and he expressed extreme doubt that they could ever encroach on the neural foramina. He also expressed his opinion as an anatomist that these changes could not possibly be of any clinical significance, with which I fully agree. He postulated further that these "calcifications" started in the ligaments around the vertebral bodies as they became lax with the aging process. As in other soft tissues in which calcium is deposited in the musculoskeletal system in life, they probably represent Nature's attempt to reinforce these weakening structures. It is quite possible that the anterior and lateral bulging of the intervertebral discs may hasten the deterioration of these ligaments, but this is probably of little clinical importance.

Even if there are osteoarthritic changes in the interlaminar and other synovial joints in the spine, characterized by the usual radiographic changes of subchondral bone sclerosis, narrowing of the joint space, and an irregularity of outline of the joint, I cannot believe that pain arises from the osteoarthritic changes, unless the cartilage is so worn away that bone rubs upon bone.

Usually, osteoarthritis is a painless change in synovial joints brought on by excess wear and tear on the articular cartilages. Certainly the space-occupying property of the articular cartilage is lessened, which therefore allows laxity in the supporting ligaments and overmovement in the joints. This results in joint

* Shore, L. R. On osteo-arthritis in the dorsal intervertebral joints. *Brit. J. Surg.*, Vol. XXII, No. 85:833, 1936.
    Shore, L. R. Polyspondylitis marginalis osteophytica. *Brit. J. Surg.*, Vol. XXII, No. 85:850, 1936.

instability, and a propensity for joint locking and joint dysfunction when such a joint is subjected to any unguarded movement during the performance of a voluntary movement. Later,
loss of elasticity in, and shrinking of, the capsule may inhibit
movement and produce dysfunction. It is surely the loss of movement, or the presence of abnormal movement stretching the joint
capsule or ligaments, which gives rise to pain. Restoration of
normal movement usually relieves the pain. Osteoarthritis is no
contraindication for manipulative therapy.

Certainly it must be conceded that if by any treatment a
painful osteoarthritic joint is relieved of its symptoms, there is
no visible alteration of the changes seen radiographically in the
joint after treatment. This strongly suggests that the osteoarthritic
changes themselves are blameless, insofar as the production of
symptoms goes.

Infective Arthritis

The spinal synovial joints may be the seat of any infective
type of arthritis, or even gout. These conditions contraindicate
manipulative therapy except, following the eradication of the
infective process, when residual joint dysfunction is still present.
When the infective process is quiescent or eradicated by suitable
treatment, the history of the pain symptom changes from an
increased stiffness following rest to a relief of symptoms after
rest.

Infective arthritides in the spine are usually referred to by
the term "infective spondylitis." They are usually secondary to
a distant focus of infection. The worst cases I have seen have
been in association with gonorrhea and acute bacterial endocarditis. A very similar clinical picture occurs with serum sick-
ness. The low grade infective spondylitis from dental sepsis

merits just as much respect in treatment. Brucellosis, tuberculosis and fungus infections of the bones and joints of the spine must never be forgotten as etiological possibilities. And a trap differential diagnosis of infective spondylitis is a tabetic crisis.

Ankylosing Spondylitis

The problem of "rheumatic" spondylitis merits discussion. Commonly referred to as Marie-Strümpell spondylitis, I prefer the diagnostic term of Gilbert Scott — "ankylosing spondylitis of adolescence." I find it very difficult to believe that this is a rheumatoid condition or the analogue in the spine of the peripheral disease — rheumatoid arthritis. This crippling disease — ankylosing spondylitis — certainly merits a great deal of further research. It is the study of the natural history of this disease which especially points up the dissimilarity between it and rheumatoid arthritis.

Whereas rheumatoid arthritis occurs chiefly in asthenic women in the third and fourth decades of life, and primarily affects the small joints of the extremities, ankylosing spondylitis occurs predominately in adolescent athletic youths and always starts in the sacroiliac joints, producing changes interpreted by radiologists as sacroiliitis, and progresses up the spine. If it attacks any of the joints of the extremities, it attacks the large joints, especially the hips and shoulders.

Ankylosis in rheumatoid arthritis, when it occurs, is fibrous and intra-articular; ankylosis in ankylosing spondylitis is bony and periarticular, the perivertebral ligaments being calcified and the discs being spared. Bony fusion occurs in the sacroiliac joints.

While both diseases may exhibit spontaneous remissions, rheumatoid arthritis does respond to treatment using salicylates, gold, protein shock therapy, sometimes to psychiatric treatment and, of course, to cortisone; it shows no response to X-ray therapy. Ankylosing spondylitis is commonly arrested by X-ray therapy (especially when given by the wide field method of Gilbert Scott* as modified by F. Hernaman-Johnson, M.D.**). It responds temporarily to cortisone therapy, but salicylates, gold, protein shock treatment and psychiatric treatment do not alter its course. Pregnancy commonly produces a remission in rheumatoid arthritis. Though ankylosing spondylitis is rare in women, when it occurs, pregnancy is usually complicated by it rather than the disease being temporarily relieved.

It is inexcusable to watch ankylosing spondylitis progressing under your eyes while treating the patient with anti-rheumatoid drugs just to avoid the potential dangers of radiation. Even though it may be true that patients treated with X-rays may eventually exhibit a relatively high incidence of leukemia, untreated patients can look forward only to the life of a complete cripple, often in constant unremitting pain. They will also be prone to upper respiratory tract infections, which so easily may prove fatal. The stasis in their lungs, because of ankylosis in the joints of their thoracic cage, is a much more certain result of inadequate therapy than the possible deleterious effects on the bone marrow as a result of X-ray treatment.

When this disease is arrested, there is an important place for manipulative therapy in restoring and maintaining movement in the unaffected joints.

Osteitis Condensans Ilii

A word of warning about making the erroneous differential diagnosis of sacroiliitis, which is the precursor of ankylosing spondylitis, instead of osteitis condensans ilii is not out of place.

---

* Scott, S. Gilbert. *Wide Field X-ray Treatment*. George Newnes Ltd., 1939.
** Hernaman-Johnson, F., and Law, W. Alexander. *Ankylosing Spondylitis*. Butterworth Medical Publications, 1949.

The latter (osteitis condensans ilii) is usually asymptomatic and an incidental finding in an X-ray examination. It is more frequently seen in parous women rather than young men and is never associated with systemic signs of disease such as an increased sedimentation rate, relative changes in the differential white cell count, night sweats, fever, and sometimes cachexia. In other words, osteitis condensans ilii, though superficially suggesting sacroiliitis radiologically, is a local benign change in the iliac bones adjacent to the sacroiliac joints. Figure 76 shows a case of osteitis condensans ilii. The points to be noted are the typical triangular shape of the abnormally sclerotic areas, the

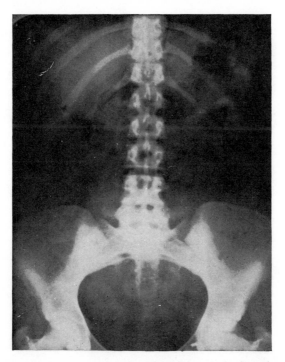

FIGURE 76. Osteitis condensans ilii. Note the typical triangular area of sclerosis confined to the iliac bones, and the clear sacroiliac spaces. This appearance should be compared with the irregular sclerosis, which involves both the sacral and the iliac bones, and the irregular sacroiliac joint spaces, parts of which cannot be distinguished, shown in Figure 77. (From the collection of D. H. Gehagen, M.D.)

changes being confined to the iliac bones adjacent to the sacroiliac joint spaces; also, the sacroiliac joint spaces are clear and
have regular margins. Figure 77 shows a case of ankylosing
spondylitis, illustrating sacroiliitis. Abnormal sclerosis is seen to
involve both the iliac bone and the adjacent sacrum; the sacroiliac joint spaces are irregular in outline, and in places cannot
be distinguished. Figure 78 shows an X-ray of a patient in which
the differential diagnosis was anything but clear, either clinically
or radiologically. The patient complained of pain and increasing
stiffness of his back, the symptoms being confirmed by clinical
signs. He was running a fever. His sedimentation rate was 62 mm.

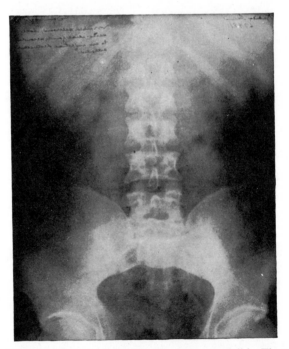

FIGURE 77.   Sacroiliitis in a case of ankylosing spondylitis. The sclerosis
involves both the sacral and iliac bones, and the sacroiliac joint spaces are
irregular and in places cannot be distinguished. Compare this figure with
Figure 76. (From the collection of R. J. Steinborg, M.D.)

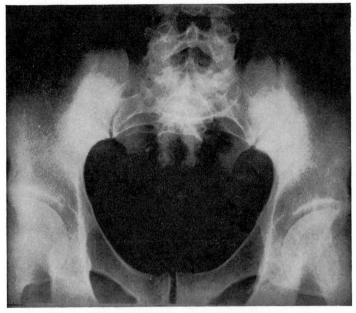

FIGURE 78.   Osteitis condensans ilii. The differential diagnosis between sacroiliitis and osteitis condensans ilii proved difficult, both clinically and radiologically. Careful study shows that the sclerosis is confined to the iliac bones and the sacroiliac joint spaces are clear. (From the collection of R. J. Steinborg, M.D.)

in the first hour. The X-ray changes are clear. However, careful study of the picture shows that the abnormal sclerosis is confined to the iliac bones and that the sacroiliac joints spaces are clear. The sedimentation rate dropped to 2 mm. in the first hour and the patient's signs of systemic disease and his symptoms of back pain and stiffness disappeared after he had received adequate treatment for his acute prostatitis. The somewhat misleading radiographic changes in the sacroiliac area remained unchanged and are due to osteitis condensans ilii.

The reader is reminded of the pathognomonic sign of sacroiliac joint disease described on page 62. In this condition there is a loss of movement between the posterior superior iliac spines with change of posture. The absence of this sign in the confusing case described above should have given the clue to the correct nature of the changes in the patient's X-rays and should always help to avoid confusing the two conditions.

I conclude, then, that osteoarthritis plays an insignificant role in the production of back pain. The other forms of arthritis are usually amenable to suitable treatment.

13

The Whiplash Injury

It was at the 1957 postgraduate Alumni Conference of the College of Medical Evangelists that I first realized the anxiety which the whiplash injury of the neck is causing in our profession.

The most common question I was asked as a scientific exhibitor at this conference was: "How do you treat whiplash injuries?" It seems that this condition has become one of the most popular medicolegal gimmicks on the West Coast. This can only mean that there is a great lack of understanding about the subject in clinical practice.

Of course, one answer to the question asked is that I do not treat whiplash injuries. The term is a lay term, descriptive of etiology, but meaningless diagnostically. The sooner it is dropped from medical jargon, the sooner the confusion which results from its use will be cleared away. Only then may patients who have suffered from such an injury expect to receive adequate care for posttraumatic symptoms in their heads, necks and arms.

Any treatment prescribed for a whiplash injury can only be empirical, or by means of trial and error. This constitutes poor medical practice, opening wide the doors for spurious medicolegal suits, which can bring only discredit to our profession.

Pathology

Correct diagnosis of the pathology underlying symptoms is a prerequisite of successful treatment. Careful clinical examination is a prerequisite of correct diagnosis.

I have drawn attention to the fact that the cervical spine is the most difficult section of the spine to examine and that the diagnosis of back pathology depends to a considerable degree on clinical inference. There can be little doubt that the whiplash injury to the neck is the most complicated injury to analyze and therefore, perhaps, the most difficult one in which inferences may be drawn. X-rays are a help only when the injury results in obvious dislocations and fractures. The laboratory cannot be of assistance.

The method of examination of these cases does not vary from that advocated in this work. The signs elicited by examination might be rather easier to interpret if there were any other anatomical structure in the more easily handled extremities which suffers the same type of injury with which these signs might be compared.

I venture to suggest that "twisting" of an "ankle" is analogous to the whiplash injury of the neck and that study of the whiplash injury of the ankle will help our understanding of the whiplash injury of the neck.

Movement in the mortise joint is pure flexion and extension and in this joint there are only two movements of joint play: long-axis extension and an anteroposterior glide of the tibial and fibular articulations on the astragalus. There is nothing very special about this to warrant the choice of the "ankle" by which to illustrate any neck movement. It is in considering the subastragaloid joint, which is all too often neglected in "ankle" injuries, that the analogy is most important.

Anatomy texts describe the voluntary movement at the subastragaloid joint as being inversion and eversion of the ankle. If that were all, this joint would be relatively unimportant, because these movements are also available to the foot at the midtarsal and metatarsophalangeal rows of joints. The most important movement at the subastragaloid joint is the involuntary movement of anteroposterior rock of the astragalus on the calcaneus; without this the astragalus would invariably dislocate when forward motion of the foot is arrested unexpectedly by stubbing the toes in some manner. The wide range in the movement of joint play of long-axis extension makes this movement the more efficient. In addition, there is a wide range in the movement of joint play of side tilt, both medially and laterally, in the absence of which fractures of the malleoli would be inevitable following even insignificant trauma.

The similarity between the astragalar rock and the occipital rock is remarkable. Dysfunction from a traumatic joint lock in the subastragaloid joint following the reduction of a dislocation or the healing of a fracture, or following disuse after plaster immobilization, produces more disability at the ankle than results from any other cause. Similarly, I believe, dysfunction at the occipito-atlantal joint produces more residual symptoms in the neck following the whiplash than result from any other cause.

There can be no controversy that the most innocuous result of a twisted "ankle" is a synovitis in the mortise or subastragaloid joint, or both. A slightly more severe injury produces hemarthrosis in one or both of these joints. Any of these conditions may be complicated by a partial ligamentous tear. When the injury is more severe, a true Pott's fracture may result (fracture in the distal third of the fibula and rupture of the medial deltoid ligament). A more severe injury produces a bi- or trimalleolar fracture; a worse one still produces similar fractures complicated by a dislocation of the astragalus; and yet a worse injury produces a fracture in which all these things occur together with a dislocation of the inferior tibiofibular joint. With the fractures and fracture dislocations there is severe swelling of the soft tissues from edema and hematomata.

There can be no doubt that a similar progression of pathological conditions affects the neck following the whiplash injury.

This is where the similarities between the ankle and neck whiplash end. Now the singular peculiarities of the neck and their relation to symptoms following injury must be considered.

In the cervical spine, there are nineteen synovial joints, the eight pairs of major interlaminar joints, the important odontoid-atlas joint and the six pairs of joints of Luschka. There are six intervertebral discs. The close proximity of the spinal cord and the cervical nerve roots to the skeletal structures which may suffer injury may produce complicating features. The cervical sympathetic ganglia may become involved in the soft tissue trauma. Other differences between the ankle and the neck which are important are that, whereas at the ankle the muscles are discretely tendinous as they pass in relation to the joints, in the neck they are both tendinous and fleshy; and the ligaments supporting the ankle are relatively resilient and discrete, whereas in the neck they are tight and cannot be differentiated. Then too, the range of movement at the ankle joints is relatively circumscribed, and when one ankle is subjected to injury, the weight which it is designed to support can be shared by the other leg, or relieved by falling before very much direct stress is imposed. In the neck the composite movement of the joints of the cervical spine results in poor stability, and the weight of the head can never be shared or removed during any part of a traumatic episode. Symptoms may arise following the whiplash injury in joints as far down the spine as the sixth thoracic vertebra, and signs of joint injury must always be looked for as far down the back as this.

A unique complication of a whiplash injury of the neck results from the close relationship to the spine of the pharynx and esophagus, and even the larynx and trachea.

Joint Lock. The most innocuous pathology of the whiplash in the neck, then, is a joint lock at any of the synovial joints. If the injury be sustained in the anteroposterior plane, this occurs at the occipito-atlantal junction, and pain from this may be felt locally and/or radiating up over the occiput into the head. Rotation and forward bending of the head on the neck may be impaired. If the injury is sustained while the head is partially rotated on the neck, any of the interlaminar joints may be locked, usually on the side away from that toward which the head was turned. The symptoms of a simple joint lock are limitation of some involuntary movement and pain at the limit of movement, either local to the joint or referred to some distant point along the segmental nerve, relieved by rest and aggravated by movement. The treatment of joint lock is the restoration of the lost movement in the range of joint play by manipulation.

Synovitis. A slightly more severe injury produces a synovitis in the interlaminar joints which are most affected by the injury. The symptoms now are some immediate discomfort in the neck at the level which is affected, followed by a period of some hours of improvement, followed by an increased stiffness and pain in the neck, often first noticed on waking next morning. If the synovial swelling becomes at all marked, irritation of the nerve root in relation to it may occur, giving the false impression of a disc lesion because of the presence of pain radiation, paresthesiae, muscle weakness, and maybe sensory and reflex changes. The differentiation may not be easy, and a lumbar puncture may have to be done before a diagnosis may be made. However, with proper treatment, the signs from synovitis rapidly disappear within a few days, whereas the signs from a prolapsed disc persist and may worsen.

The proper treatment for synovitis is rest of the involved joint from function but movement of the joint and its supporting muscles without function. Specifically, rest by means of a temporary Thomas collar, intermittent traction, preferably with the patient sitting upright, and the application of heat three or four times a day should be the treatment program. If available, anodal iontophoresis has a pain-relieving effect, either of its own or following Novocain infiltration. It also tends to increase the flow of edema fluid away from the electrode, thereby assisting the dissipation of the swelling by increasing the permeability of the synovial membrane by chemicophysical means. Some degree of joint dysfunction may remain following resolution of the synovitis, and the patient will not be free of pain until full normal movement has been restored. The indication of clearing synovitis but residual dysfunction is a change of symptoms from stiffening with rest to a relief from discomfort following rest, but recurrence of pain following activity.

Hemarthrosis. A still more severe injury results in a hemarthrosis. The symptoms are acute local pain with loss of movement, tending to worsen in the first few hours following the injury. Differentiation of this condition clinically from a fracture or dislocation can only be achieved by the absence of X-ray evidence of bone or joint injury. The correct treatment of a hemarthrosis is aspiration of the involved joint. This is technically impossible in the interlaminar joints of the spine, so immobilization by continuous traction, sedation, and the application of ice is the best treatment available in the acute stage. Once the acute stage has passed, treatment such as that used for synovitis is instituted and any residual dysfunction, which in this instance is probably due to intra-articular adhesions, must be overcome by manipulation. There is often a synovial joint reaction when adhesions are torn, and this in turn requires a period of appropriate physical therapy, in addition to maintaining the range of movement restored each day until the therapeutic reaction is quiescent.

Any of the above three pathological conditions may occur singly. With any severe injury, more than one pathological condition will occur, and each must be treated before the patient can be expected to be relieved of his symptoms.

Soft Tissue Injury. The next thing that may happen in order of severity of the injury is tearing of the supporting soft tissues of the neck, first the muscles and then the ligaments, particularly the interspinous ligaments. Severe soft tissue injury may be associated with hemorrhage into the retropharyngeal space, and when this occurs it takes precedence in treatment. Embarrassment of respiration may make this an acute surgical emergency. Embarrassment of deglutition may require intravenous feeding.

Having dealt with these complications as indicated, the treatment of a muscle tear must be undertaken. Whereas the treatment of hemorrhage includes the application of ice, this should now be changed to the application of heat. Whereas immobilization is part of the treatment of hemorrhage, this should now be changed to movement of the damaged muscle by exercises of it without use. This is best achieved by the use of faradic stimulation using the Smart-Bristow Coil. The intensity and the frequency of the current should be graduated by the therapist, the indication for increasing the treatment being the absence of pain. The heat and faradism must be followed by light stroking massage (effleurage) to attain muscle relaxation and to disperse any congestion remaining from the application of heat. The symptoms and signs of a muscle tear are muscle spasm, inaccurately localized pain, and stiffening of the neck with rest. There is local acute tenderness in the muscle on palpation, as well as a feeling of a gathering of the torn muscle fibers. Infiltration of the torn area with Novacain, followed by ionization, may be necessary before the more active physical therapy is started.

A torn joint ligament can scarcely be present without a torn muscle. A ligament tear requires a longer period of immobilization for healing to take place. The diagnosis is not easy, but tension on the ligament by passive movement without muscle stretch produces pain. A tear in an interspinous ligament can be detected on palpation by eliciting acute tenderness localized between two spinous processes.

A ruptured interlaminar joint ligament must be clinically hypothetical, but the condition does occur and can be recognized at surgery. Persistent or frequently recurring local pain from continuing joint instability always in the same place should suggest this possibility. A ruptured interspinous ligament is detected by the presence of a dip on palpation between two spinous processes and signs of intervertebral junction instability. I have seen one case each of these ruptured ligaments and the only effective treatment was spine fusion at the affected junction.

An injury of similar severity may result in avulsion of a part of a spinous process without rupture of the attached ligament. I have only seen this at the sixth and seventh cervical vertebrae following a whiplash injury. Treatment by immobilization until the patient is symptom-free, followed by treatment of residual muscle pathology or joint dysfunction, is sufficient in these cases.

Dislocation and Fracture. An injury of about the same severity may produce dislocation of a facet joint. This can be detected radiologically and should promptly be reduced, the aftertreatment being the same as for any other dislocated weight-bearing joint.

An injury of any greater severity produces a vertebral body fracture, with or without dislocation; complications may be serious and treatment very prolonged. An acute prolapse of a disc may occur. An epidural hematoma may form. The anterior spinal artery may be traumatized, resulting in myelomalacia. There may be a transient cord concussion. There may be cord severance. Treatment of these conditions lies in the specialist fields and will not be discussed here. But there should never be any reluctance to perform a lumbar puncture with manometric studies and determination of the protein and cellular content in the diagnostic work-up of patients following a whiplash injury. The examination of the patient must always include study of the nervous system.

Residual Symptoms — Treatment

The important thing is how to assess residual symptoms once recovery from these severe pathological conditions has occurred. We must ignore residual quadriplegia, which requires prolonged rehabilitation techniques, and confine ourselves to local pain in the neck and pain referred from the neck.

The only basis on which residual symptoms can be assessed is adequate clinical examination. The common causes of residual symptoms are simple untreated joint dysfunction with or without pain referred into the head, joint dysfunction due to intra-articular adhesions, adherent scar formation in the supporting muscles of the neck, unhealed ligament pathology resulting in joint or junction instability, irreversible disc pathology, muscle imbalance or weakness due to atrophy from prolonged spasm or transient paresis, or any mixture of any of the above causes. The conditions can be differentiated clinically and treated specifically and successfully. Seldom, in my experience, are residual symptoms psychogenic. Usually there is a physical basis for residual symptoms. Any psychological overlay usually is a direct result of the failure to diagnose and to relieve successfully the patient of his symptoms, which may result in the development of a fear of permanent disability. The psychological aspect can only be successfully treated by removal of the physical cause. The physical disability can never be removed by psychological treatment, tranquilizers or pain-killing drugs.

There is no doubt that residual symptoms often result from some autonomic dysfunction. I believe that the most likely mechanism of this is an irritation of the cervicothoracic or stellate sympathetic ganglia, either by pressure from local swelling due to blood or edema or reflexly because of irritation of the nerve roots (particularly the first and second thoracic nerves) with which the ganglion is connected by its *rami communicantes.*

Symptoms and signs which direct one's attention to the stellate ganglion are causalgic shoulder and arm pain, trophic skin changes, especially of the hands and fingers, swelling and stiffness of the hands, excess palmar perspiration, dilatation of the ipsilateral pupil and the palpebral fissure, proptosis with oculopalpebral asynergia, and deficient convergence of the eyeballs. The arm symptoms and signs are common; the gross eye signs are not.

Treatment by stellate ganglion block often brings dramatic

relief, especially of the arm pains and the changes in the hands.

Vertigo is another residual symptom of which sufferers from the whiplash injury may complain. Body equilibrium is co-ordinated in the cerebellum from impulses from the labyrinth, the inner ear, the eyes, the skin, the muscles and the joints. Maintenance of equilibrium is regulated by the cerebellum and is largely a muscular effect, influenced by the activity of the tonic neck reflexes among other things. Equilibrium can be affected by dysfunction in the joints and spasm in the muscles of the neck. Treatment of posttraumatic vertigo may well include mobilization of the joints of the cervical spine.

Residual pain in the neck may arise from nonunion or fibrous union in fractures which have been overlooked, and therefore not treated. These may occur in the laminae, at the base of the odontoid process of the axis or, I suspect, in the exterior facets of the joints of Luschka. Treatment of these complications will probably have to be surgical, either by neurectomy, rhizotomy, or spine fusion.

I am sure that residual symptoms from the whiplash injury of the neck would be nonexistent, or at least minimal, if the treatment of the pathology resulting from it were instituted from the time of the injury.

14

Conclusion

I hope that this work will help to clarify the status of joint manipulation in its relationship to the diagnosis of pain arising in and from synovial joints and to the treatment for relief of common distressing symptoms.

I hope that many of my colleagues, who from personal experience know how much benefit may be derived from manipulation of the spinal joints, will be encouraged to support my advocacy that this subject should promptly receive attention both in medical schools and postgraduate training programs.

The basic deficiencies in our understanding of the common simple back problem are educational. This is largely because of the biased or uninformed opinions of a vociferous minority which for years have been directed against groups of practitioners who are not medically qualified but for the most part simply share our wish to bring comfort as quickly and efficiently as possible to those who are suffering from pain. It is unfortunate, then, that the altruistic aims of the majority have been lost in the confusion of the politics of the minority. I would encourage those in our profession carefully to examine and follow up patients who have derived benefit from manipulation, and to decide for themselves upon its merits. Doctors of Medicine are particularly fortunate in their trained ability for critique, and should welcome into their ever-widening armamentarium of medical practice all that is good in manipulative practice.

With such support from within our profession, and with continued pressure from the demands of our patients, I believe that in the foreseeable future manipulation will be, and should be, as readily forthcoming from the family physician as a diathermy treatment (which at best can only be comforting and palliative) or a pain pill (which may be deluding). Certainly, until patients find more sure and prompt relief from their back symptoms they will continue to develop the haunting anxieties, both economic and emotional, which are currently concomitant with all forms of back pain. Such anxieties detract from good relations between us.

I wish I could say that manipulative therapy is the only modality of physical treatment that need be learned to bring relief from ubiquitous backache. Often it is. But just as often it is necessary to use other modalities as well before the patient can obtain relief. However, there are about 8000 trained physical therapists throughout this country, available expertly to administer adequately prescribed physical therapy. It is necessary to learn what is available and then how to prescribe what is necessary.

Certainly for a population of 175 million there should be, at a conservative estimate, about 60,000 trained physical therapists to fill the needs of doctors and their patients. But, until physicians are taught, and learn the wide uses of physical treatment in every branch of medicine (as well as in the orthopaedic and physical medicine fields), the profession of a physical therapist will remain unattractive and, because of lack of trained personnel, the public will continue to be deprived of the benefits of these treatment modalities for some time to come.

This work will draw attention to a wide gap in medical knowledge. I hope it will encourage many to start to try to bridge the gap.

Meanwhile, if you can satisfy yourself that a patient's symptoms are arising from joint dysfunction, then I think you are justified in asking a well-trained manipulator, whoever he may be, to treat your patient for that specific complaint, just as you would ask a radiographer to take an X-ray picture, or a laboratory technician to do a blood examination, or a pharmacist to make up a prescription.

But you must make the diagnosis yourself and be prepared to take the responsibility for the treatment you prescribe.

I must conclude with an admonition: Learn well what to do, and how and when to do it, before personally attempting therapeutic manipulation; but do not deprive your patients of relief from pain because of your prejudice.

Index